1 Pharmacokinetics	2 What does "pharmacokinetics" include?
3 The main mechanism of most drugs absorption in GI tract is	4 What kind of substances can't permeate membranes by passive diffusion?
5 A hydrophilic medicinal agent has the following property	6 What is implied by «active transport»?
7 What does the term "bioavailability" mean?	8 The reasons determing bioavailability are
9 Pick out the appropriate alimentary route of administration when passage of drugs through liver is minimized	10 Which route of drug administration is most likely to lead to the first-pass effect?

1 The study of absorption, distribution, metabolism and excretion of drugs.	2 - Drug biotransformation in the organism- Distribution of drugs in the organism- Excretion of substances
3 Passive diffusion (lipid diffusion)	4 Hydrophilic substances
5 Low ability to penetrate through the cell membrane lipids.	6 Transport against concentration gradient
7 Fraction of an uncharged drug reaching the systemic circulation following any route administration.	8 Extent of absorption and hepatic first-pass effect
9 Rectal	10 Oral

1
What is characteristic of the oral route?

2
Tick the feature of the sublingual route

3
Pick out the parenteral route of medicinal agent administration

4
Parenteral administration

5
What is characteristic of the intramuscular route of drug administration?

6
True or False. Intravenous injections are more suitable for oily solutions.

7
True or False. Intravenous administration provides a rapid response

8
True or False. Intramuscular administration requires a sterile technique

9
True or False. Subcutaneous administration may cause local irritation

10
True or False. Most of drugs are distributed homogeneously.

1 Absorption depends on GI tract secretion and motor function.	2 Pretty fast absorption
3 Inhalation, IV.	4 Usually produces a more rapid response than oral administration
5 Oily solutions can be injected	6 FALSE.
7 TRUE	8 TRUE
9 TRUE	10 FALSE

1 Biological barriers include	**2** What is the reason of complicated penetration of some drugs through brain-blood barrier?
3 The volume of distribution (Vd) relates	**4** For the calculation of the volume of distribution (Vd) one must take into account
5 The term "biotransformation" includes	**6** Tick the drug type for which microsomal oxidation is the most prominent
7 True or False. Microsomal oxidation results in an increase of ionization and water solubility of a drug	**8** Stimulation of liver microsomal enzymes can
9 Metabolic transformation (phase 1) is	**10** Biotransformation of a medicinal substance results in

1 - Cell membranes- Capillary walls- Placenta	2 Absence of pores in the brain capillary endothelium
3 The amount of a drug in the body to the concentration of a drug in plasma.	4 Concentration of a substance in plasma
5 Process of physicochemical and biochemical alteration of a drug in the body.	6 Lipid soluble
7 TRUE	8 Require the dose increase of some drugs.
9 Transformation of substances due to oxidation, reduction or hydrolysis.	10 Faster urinary excretion.

1

Conjugation

2

Which of the following processes proceeds in the second phase of biotransformation

3

Conjugation of a drug includes

4

True or False. Metabolic transformation and conjugation usually results in an increase of a substance biological activity

5

In case of liver disorders accompanied by a decline in microsomal enzyme activity the duration of action of some drugs is

6

Half life (t ½) is the time required to

7

Half life (t ½) doesn't depend on

8

Half life (t ½) depends on

9

Elimination is expressed as

10

Elimination rate constant (Kelim) is defined by the following parameter

1	2
Coupling of a drug with an endogenous substrate	Acetylation

3	4
- Glucoronidation- Sulfate formation- Methylation	FALSE

5	6
Enlarged	Change the amount of a drug in plasma by half during elimination.

7	8
Time of drug absorption	- Biotransformation- Concentration of a drug in plasma- Rate of drug elimination

9	10
Clearance of an organism from a xenobiotic.	Half life (t ½)

1. True or False. The most rapid eliminated drugs are those with high glomerular filtration rate and actively secreted but aren't passively reabsorbed

2. Systemic clearance (CLs) is related with

3. Pharmacodynamics involves the study of

4. The most appropriate to the term "receptor"

5. What does "affinity" mean

6. Target proteins which a drug molecule binds are

7. An agonist is a substance that

8. If an agonist can produce maximal effects and has high efficacy it's called

9. If an agonist can produce submaximal effects and has moderate efficacy it's called

10. An antagonist is a substance that

1	2
TRUE	Volume of distribution, half life and elimination rate constant.

3	4
- Biological and therapeutic effects of drugs- Mechanisms of drug action- Drug interactions- Information about unwanted effects	Active macromolecular components of a cell or an organism which a drug molecule has to combine with in order to elicit its specific effect

5	6
A measure of how tightly a drug binds to a receptor	- Only receptors- Only ion channels- Only carriers

7	8
Interacts with the receptor and initiates changes in cell function, producing various effects	Full agonist

9	10
Partial agonist	Binds to the receptors without directly altering their functions

1	2
A competitive antagonist is a substance that	The substance binding to one receptor subtype as an agonist and to another as an antagonist is called
3	4
Irreversible interaction of an antagonist with a receptor is due to	Tick the second messenger of G-protein-coupled (metabotropic) receptor
5	6
Tick the substance which changes the activity of an effector element but doesn't belong to second messengers	The increase of second messengers' (cAMP, cGMP, Ca^{2+} etc.) concentration leads to
7	8
Tick the substances whose mechanisms are based on interaction with ion channels	Efficacy
9	10
Potency	Therapeutical dose

1 Binds to the same receptor site and progressively inhibits the agonist response	**2** Agonist-antagonist
3 Covalent bonds	**4** cAMP
5 G–protein	**6** Proteinkinases activation and protein phosphorylation.
7 - Sodium channel blockers- Calcium channel blockers- Potassium channels activators	**8** is the maximum effect of a drug
9 is a comparative measure, refers to the different doses of two drugs that are needed to produce the same effect	**10** The amount of a substance to produce the required effect in most patients

1 Toxic dose	**2** Which effect may lead to toxic reactions when a drug is taken continuously or repeatedly
3 What term is used to describe a more gradual decrease in responsiveness to a drug, taking days or weeks to develop?	**4** What term is used to describe a decrease in responsiveness to a drug which develops in a few minutes?
5 Tachyphylaxis	**6** True or False. Drug resistance is a term used to describe the loss of effectiveness of antimicrobial or antitumour drugs.
7 Tolerance and drug resistance can be a consequence of	**8** True or False. Dependence is often associated with tolerance to a drug, a physical abstinence syndrome, and psychological dependence (craving).
9 The situation when failure to continue administering the drug results in serious psychological and somatic disturbances is called?	**10** What is the type of drug-to-drug interaction which is connected with processes of absorption, biotransformation, distribution and excretion?

1 The amount of substance to produce effects hazardous for an organism	2 Cumulative effect
3 Tolerance	4 Tachyphylaxis
5 Very rapidly developing tolerance	6 TRUE
7 - Increased metabolic degradation- Change in receptors, loss of them or exhaustion of mediators-	8 TRUE
9 Abstinence syndrome	10 Pharmacokinetic interaction

1. What is the type of drug-to-drug interaction which is the result of interaction at receptor, cell, enzyme or organ level?

2. What phenomenon can occur in case of using a combination of drugs?

3. If two drugs with the same effect, taken together, produce an effect that is equal in magnitude to the sum of the effects of the drugs given individually, it is called as

4. What does the term "potentiation" mean?

5. The types of antagonism are

6. The term "chemical antagonism" means that

7. A teratogenic action is

8. Characteristic unwanted reaction which isn't related to a dose or to a pharmacodynamic property of a drug is called

9. Idiosyncratic reaction of a drug is

10. Therapeutic index (TI) is

1	2
Pharmacodynamic interaction	Synergism

3	4
Additive effect	Intensive increase of drug effects due to their combination

5	6
Competitive	Two drugs combine with one another to form an inactive compound

7	8
Negative action on the fetus causing fetal malformation	Hypersensitivity

9	10
Unpredictable, inherent, qualitatively abnormal reaction to a drug	A ratio used to evaluate the safety and usefulness of a drug for indication

1. Local anesthetics produce

2. A good local anesthetic agent shouldn't cause

3. Most local anesthetic agents consist of

4. Which one of the following groups is responsible for the duration of the local anesthetic action?

5. Indicate the local anesthetic agent, which has a shorter duration of action

6. Which one of the following groups is responsible for the potency and the toxicity of local anesthetics?

7. Indicate the drug, which has greater potency of the local anesthetic action

8. Ionizable group is responsible for

9. Which one of the following local anesthetics is an ester of benzoic acid?

10. Indicate the local anesthetic, which is an ester of paraaminobenzoic acid

1 Blocking pain sensation without loss of consciousness	2 Fast onset and long duration of action
3 - Lipophylic group (frequently an aromatic ring)- Intermediate chain (commonly including an ester or amide)- Amino group	4 Intermediate chain
5 Procaine	6 Lipophylic group
7 Bupivacaine	8 The ability to diffuse to the site of action
9 Cocaine	10 Procaine

1. Which of the following local anesthetics is an acetanilide derivative?

2. Indicate the local anesthetic, which is a toluidine derivative

3. Which of the following local anesthetics is a thiophene derivative?

4. Local anesthetics are

5. For therapeutic application local anesthetics are usually made available as salts for the reasons of

6. Which of the following statements is not correct for local anesthetics?

7. Which one of the following statements about the metabolism of local anesthetics is incorrect?

8. Indicate the anesthetic agent of choice in patient with a liver disease

9. Which of the following local anesthetics is preferable in patient with pseudocholinesterase deficiency?

10. The primary mechanism of action of local anesthetics is

1 Lidocaine	2 Prilocaine
3 Ultracaine	4 Weak bases
5 More stability and greater water solubility	6 charged cationic form penetrates biologic membranes more readily than an uncharged form
7 Metabolism of local anesthetics occurs at the site of administration	8 Procaine
9 Ropivacaine	10 Blockade of voltage-gated sodium channels

1	2
A local anesthetics that is water-soluble	Indicate the local anesthetic, which is more lipid-soluble
3	4
The more lipophylic drugs	Which fibers is the first to be blocked?
5	6
The function, which the last to be blocked:	Which of the following fibers participates in high-frequency pain transmission?
7	8
Local anesthetics that is an useful antiarrhythmic agent?	Indicate the route of local anesthetic administration, which is associated with instillation within epidural or subarachnoid spaces
9	10
The choice of a local anesthetic for specific procedures is usually based on	What anesthetics has a short-acting drug?

1 Procaine	2 Bupivacaine
3 - Are more potent- Have longer duration of action- Bind more extensively to proteins	4 B and C fibers
5 Motor function	6 Type A delta and C fibers
7 Lidocaine	8 Spinal anesthesia
9 - The duration of action- Water solubility- Capability of rapid penetration through the skin or mucosa with limited tendency to diffuse away from the site of application	10 Procaine

1. Indicate the local anesthetic, which is a long-acting agent	2. The anesthetic effect of the agents of short and intermediate duration of action can not be prolonged by adding
3. A vasoconstrictor does not	4. A vasoconstrictor does
5. Vasoconstrictors are less effective in prolonging anesthetic properties of	6. Which of the following local anesthetics is only used for surface or topical anesthesia?
7. Indicate the local anesthetic, which is mainly used for regional nerve block anesthesia	8. Which local anesthetics is used for infiltrative and regional anesthesia?
9. Indicate the local anesthetic, which is used for spinal anesthesia	10. Which local anesthetics is called a universal anesthetic?

1	2
Bupivacaine	Dopamine

3	4
Reduce a local anesthetic uptake by the nerve	- Retard the removal of drug from the injection site- Hence the chance of toxicity- Decrease the blood level

5	6
Bupivacaine	Cocaine

7	8
Bupivacaine	- Procaine- Lidocaine- Mepivacaine

9	10
Tetracaine	Lidocaine

1. Most serious toxic reaction to local anesthetics is

2. Correct statements concerning cocaine include

3. Which local anesthetics is more cardiotoxic?

4. Most local anesthetics can cause

5. Which local anesthetics causes methemoglobinemia?

6. Procaine has all of the following propertie

7. Procaine has all of the following properties **EXCEPT**

8. Correct statements concerning lidocaine include

9. Correct statements concerning lidocaine include all of the following **EXCEPT**

10. Which local anesthetics is more likely to cause allergic reactions?

1	2
- Seizures- Cardiovascular collapse- Respiratory failure	- Cocaine is often used for nose and throat procedures- Limited use because of abuse potential- Causes sympathetically mediated tachycardia and vasoconstriction
3	4
Bupivacaine	- Depression of abnormal cardiac pacemaker activity, excitability, conduction- Depression of the strength of cardiac contraction- Cardiovascular collapse
5	6
Prilocaine	- It has ester linkage- Its metabolic product can inhibit the action of sulfonamides- It is relatively short-acting
7	8
It readily penetrates the skin and mucosa	- It is an universal anesthetic- It widely used as an antiarrhythmic agent- It is metabolized in liver
9	10
It has esteratic linkage	Procaine

1

Tetracaine has all of the following properties

2

Tetracaine has all of the following properties EXCEPT

3

Correct statements concerning bupivacaine include

4

Correct statements concerning bupivacaine include all of the following EXCEPT

5

Acetylcholine is not a specific neurotransmitter at

6

Acetylcholine is a specific neurotransmitter at

7

Muscarinic receptors are located in

8

Indicate the location of M2 cholinoreceptor type

9

The symptoms of mushroom poisoning include

10

The symptoms of mushroom poisoning include all of the following EXCEPT

1	2
- Slow onset- Long duration- High toxicity	Low potency
3	4
- It has amide linkage- It is a long-acting drug- An intravenous injection can lead to seizures	It has low cardiotoxicity
5	6
Sympathetic postganglionic nerve endings	- Sympathetic ganglia- Parasympathetic ganglia- Parasympathetic postganglionic nerve endings
7	8
Autonomic effector cells	Heart
9	10
- Salivation, lacrimation, nausea, vomiting- Headache, abdominal colic- Bradycardia, hypotension and shock	Dryness of mouth, hyperpyrexia, hallucination

1. Which cholinomimetics activates both muscarinic and nicotinic receptors?

2. Indicate a cholinomimetic agent, which is related to direct-acting drugs

3. Characteristics of carbachol include

4. Characteristics of carbachol include all of the following EXCEPT

5. Acetylcholine is not used in clinical practice because

6. Parasympathomimetic drugs cause

7. Which direct-acting cholinomimetics is mainly muscarinic in action?

8. Which direct-acting cholinomimetics has the shortest duration of action?

9. Bethanechol has all of the following properties

10. Bethanechol has all of the following properties EXCEPT

1	2
Bethanechol	Carbachol

3	4
- It decreases intraocular pressure- It exerts both nicotinic and muscarinic effects- It is resistant to acethylcholiesterase	It causes mydriasis

5	6
It is very rapidly hydrolyzed.	Bradycardia

7	8
Bethanechol	Acetylcholine

9	10
- It is extremely resistant to hydrolysis- Purely muscarinic in its action- It is used for abdominal urinary bladder distention	It exerts both nicotinic and muscarinic effects

1 A M-cholinimimetic agent is	2 Characteristics of pilocarpine include
3 Characteristics of pilocarpine include all of the following EXCEPT	4 Which cholinomimetics is a plant derivative with lower potency than nicotine but with a similar spectrum of action?
5 Which cholinomimetics is indirect-acting?	6 The mechanism of action of indirect-acting cholinomimetic agents is
7 Indicate a reversible cholinesterase inhibitor	8 Which cholinesterase inhibitors is irreversible?
9 Indicate cholinesterase activator	10 Isofluorophate increases all of the following effects except

1 Pilocarpine	2 - It is a tertiary amine alkaloid- It causes miosis and a decrease in intraocular pressure- It is useful in the treatment of glaucoma
3 Causes a decrease in secretory and motor activity of gut	4 Lobeline
5 Edrophonium	6 Inhibition of the hydrolysis of endogenous acetylcholine
7 Physostigmine	8 Isoflurophate
9 Pralidoxime	10 Bronchodilation

1. Isofluorophate increases all of the following effects

2. Indicate a cholinesterase inhibitor, which has an additional direct nicotinic agonist effect

3. Cholinesterase inhibitors do not produce

4. Which cholinomimetics is commonly used in the treatment of glaucoma?

5. Indicate the organophosphate cholinesterase inhibitor, which can be made up in an aqueous solution for ophthalmic use and retains its activity within a week:

6. Which cholinomimetics is most widely used for paralytic ileus and atony of the urinary bladder?

7. Chronic long-term therapy of myasthenia is usually accomplished with

8. Which cholinomimetics is a drug of choice for reversing the effects of nondepolarizing neuromuscular relaxants?

9. Indicate the reversible cholinesterase inhibitor, which penetrates the blood-brain bar

10. Which cholinomimetics is used in the treatment of atropine intoxication?

1 - Lacrimation- Muscle twitching- Salivation	2 Neostigmine
3 Dramatic hypertension and tachycardia	4 Pilocarpine
5 Echothiophate	6 Neostigmine
7 Neostigmine	8 Edrophonium
9 Physostigmine	10 Physostigmine

1

The symptoms of excessive stimulation of muscarinic receptors include

2

The symptoms of excessive stimulation of muscarinic receptors include all of the following EXCEPT

3

The excessive stimulation of muscarinic receptors by pilocarpine and choline esters is blocked competitively by:

4

The toxic effects of a large dose of nicotine include

5

The toxic effects of a large dose of nicotine include all of the following EXCEPT

6

The dominant initial sights of acute cholinesterase inhibitors intoxication include

7

The dominant initial sights of acute cholinesterase inhibitors intoxication include all of the following except

8

Which drugs is used for acute toxic effects of organophosphate cholinesterase inhibitors?

9

The group of nicotinic receptor-blocking drugs consists of

10

M3 receptor subtype is located

1	2
- Abdominal cramps, diarrhea- Increased salivation, excessive bronchial secretion- Miosis, bradycardia	Weakness of all skeletal muscles
3	4
Atropine	- Convulsions, coma and respiratory arrest- Skeletal muscle depolarization blockade and respiratory paralysis- Hypertension and cardiac arrhythmias
5	6
Hypotension and bradycardia	- Salivation, sweating- Bronchial constriction- Vomiting and diarrhea
7	8
Mydriasis	Pralidoxime
9	10
- Ganglion-blockers- Neuromuscular junction blockers	On effector cell membranes of glandular and smooth muscle cells

1. Which drugs is both a muscarinic and nicotinic blocker?

2. Indicate a muscarinic receptor-blocking drug

3. Which agents is a ganglion-blocking drug?

4. Indicate the skeletal muscle relaxant, which is a depolarizing agent

5. Which drugs is a nondepolarizing muscle relaxant?

6. Indicate the drug, which is rapidly and fully distributed into CNS and has a greater effect than most other antimuscarinic agents?

7. The effect of the drug on parasympathetic function declines rapidly in

8. The effect of the drug on parasympathetic function declines rapidly in all organs EXCEPT

9. The mechanism of atropine action is

10. The tissues most sensitive to atropine are

1 Benztropine	2 Scopolamine
3 Hexamethonium	4 Succinylcholine
5 Pancuronium	6 Scopolamine
7 - Heart- Smooth muscle organs- Glands	8 Eye
9 Competitive muscarinic blockade	10 The salivary, bronchial and sweat glands

1	2
Atropine is highly selective for	Which antimuscarinic drugs is often effective in preventing or reversing vestibular disturbances, especially motion sickness?
3	4
Atropine causes	Patients complain of dry or "sandy" eyes when receiving large doses of
5	6
All of the following parts of the heart are very sensitive to muscarinic receptor blockade	All of the following parts of the heart are very sensitive to muscarinic receptor blockade except:
7	8
Atropine causes	Atropine is frequently used prior to administration of inhalant anesthetics to reduce
9	10
Atropine is now rarely used for the treatment of peptic ulcer because of	Which antimuscarinic drugs is a selective M1 blocker?

1	2
- M1 receptor subtype- M2 receptor subtype- M3 receptor subtype	Scopolamine
3	4
Mydriasis, a rise in intraocular pressure and cyclo	Atropine
5	6
- Atria- Sinoatrial node- Atrioventricular node	Ventricle
7	8
Tachycardia, little effect on blood pressure and bronchodilation	Secretions
9	10
- Slow gastric empting and prolongation of the exposure of the ulcer bed to acid- Low efficiency and necessity of large doses- Adverse effects	Pirenzepine

1 Atropine causes	**2** Which drugs is useful in the treatment of uterine spasms?
3 Atropine may cause a rise in body temperature (atropine fever)	**4** The pharmacologic actions of scopolamine most closely resemble those of
5 Compared with atropine, scopolamine has all of the following properties	**6** Compared with atropine, scopolamine has all of the following properties EXCEPT
7 Which drugs is useful in the treatment of Parkinson's disease?	**8** Indicate the antimuscarinic drug, which is used as a mydriatic
9 Which agents is used as an inhalation drug in asthma?	**10** Which agents is most effective in regenerating cholinesterase associated with skeletal muscle neuromuscular junctions?

1	2
Spasmolitic activity	Atropine

3	4
In infants and children	Atropine

5	6
- More marked central effect - More potent in producing mydriasis and cycloplegia - Lower effects on the heart, bronchial muscle and intestines	Less potent in decreasing bronchial salivary and sweat gland secretion

7	8
Benztropine	Homatropine

9	10
Ipratropium	Pralidoxime

1. Indicate an antimuscarinic drug, which is effective in the treatment of mushroom poising

2. Antimuscarinics are used in the treatment of

3. Antimuscarinics are used in the treatment of the following disorders EXCEPT

4. The atropine poisoning includes all of the following symptoms EXCEPT

5. The atropine poisoning includes all of the following symptoms

6. The treatment of the antimuscarinic effects can be carried out with

7. Contraindications to the use of antimuscarinic drugs are

8. Contraindications to the use of antimuscarinic drugs are all of the following except

9. Hexamethonium blocks the action of acetylcholine and similar agonists at

10. The applications of the ganglion blockers have disappeared because of all of the following reasons EXCEPT

1	2
Atropine	- Motion sickness- Hyperhidrosis- Asthma
3	4
Glaucoma	Bradicardia, orthostatic hypotension
5	6
- Mydriasis, cycloplegia- Hyperthermia, dry mouth, hot and flushed skin- Agitation and delirium	Neostigmine
7	8
- Glaucoma- Myasthenia- Paralytic ileus and atony of the urinary bladder	Bronchial asthma
9	10
Autonomic ganglia	Respiratory depression

1. The applications of the ganglion blockers have disappeared because of all of the following reasons

2. Which agents is a short-acting ganglion blocker?

3. Indicate the ganglion-blocking drug, which can be taken orally for the treatment of hypertension?

4. The systemic effects of hexamethonium include

5. The systemic effects of hexamethonium include all of the following EXCEPT

6. Ganglion blocking drugs are used for the following emergencies

7. Ganglion blocking drugs are used for the following emergencies EXCEPT

8. Agents that produce neuromuscular blockade act by inhibiting:

9. Skeletal muscle relaxation and paralysis can occur from interruption of functions at several sites, including

10. Skeletal muscle relaxation and paralysis can occur from interruption of functions at several sites, including all of the following EXCEPT

1 - Orthostatic hypotension- Lack of selectivity- Homeostatic reflexes block	**2** Trimethaphane
3 Mecamylamine	**4** - Reduction of both peripheral vascular resistance and venous return- Partial mydriasis and loss of accommodation- Constipation and urinary retention
5 Stimulation of thermoregulatory sweating	**6** - Hypertensive crises- Controlled hypotension- Pulmonary edema
7 Cardiovascular collapse	**8** Interaction of acetylcholine with cholinergic receptors
9 - Nicotinic acetylcholine receptors- The motor end plate- Contractile apparatus	**10** Muscarinic acetylcholine receptors

1. Nondepolarisation neuromuscular blocking agents

2. Which drugs has "double-acetylcholine" structure?

3. Indicate the long-acting neuromuscular blocking agent

4. Which neuromuscular blocking drugs is an intermediate-duration muscle relaxant?

5. Indicate the nondepolarizing agent, which has the fastest onset of effect?

6. Indicate the neuromuscular blocker, whose breakdown product readily crosses the blood-brain barrier and may cause seizures

7. Which competitive neuromuscular blocking agent could be used in patients with renal failure?

8. Indicate the nondepolarizing agent, which has short duration of action

9. Which depolarizing agent has the extremely brief duration of action?

10. Neuromuscular blockade by both succinylcholine and mivacurium may be prolonged in patients wit

1 Prevent access of the transmitter to its receptor and depolarization	2 Succylcholine
3 Tubocurarine	4 Vecuronium
5 Rapacuronium	6 Atracurium
7 Atracurium	8 Mivacurium
9 Succinylcholine	10 - An abnormal variant of plasma cholinesterase- Hepatic disease

1. Depolarizing agents include all of the following properties EXCEPT

2. Which neuromuscular blockers causes transient muscle fasciculations?

3. Indicate muscles, which are more resistant to block and recover more rapidly

4. Which neuromuscular blocking agent has the potential to cause the greatest release of histamine?

5. Which of the following muscular relaxants causes hypotension and bronchospasm?

6. Indicate the neuromuscular blocker, which causes tachycardia

7. Which neuromuscular blocking agents cause cardiac arrhythmias?

8. Effects seen only with depolarizing blockade include

9. Effects seen only with depolarizing blockade include all of the following EXCEPT

10. Which neuromuscular blocking agent is contraindicated in patients with glaucoma?

1	2
Interact with nicotinic receptor to compete with acetylcholine without receptor activation	Succinylcholine

3	4
Diaphragm	Tubocurarine

5	6
Tubocurarine	Pancuronium

7	8
Succinylcholine	- Hypercaliemia- Emesis- Muscle pain

9	10
A decrease in intraocular pressure	Succinylcholine

1. Indicate the following neuromuscular blocker, which would be contraindicated in patients with renal failure

2. All of the following drugs increase the effects of depolarizing neuromuscular blocking agents EXCEPT

3. Drugs that increase the effects of depolarizing neuromuscular blocking agents

4. Which diseases can augment the neuromuscular blockade produced by nondepolarizing muscle relaxants?

5. Indicate the agent, which effectively antagonizes the neuromuscular blockade caused by nondepolarizing drugs

6. Sympathetic stimulation is mediated by

7. Characteristics of epinephrine include

8. Characteristics of epinephrine include all of the following EXCEPT

9. Which of the following sympathomimetics acts indirectly?

10. Indirect action includes all of the following properties EXCEPT

1	2
Pipecuronium	Nondepolarizing blockers

3	4
- Aminoglycosides- Antiarrhythmic drugs- Local anesthetics	Myasthenia gravis

5	6
Neostigmine	- Release of norepinephrine from nerve terminals- Activation of adrenoreceptors on postsynaptic sites- Release of epinephrine from the adrenal medulla

7	8
- It is synthesized into the adrenal medulla- It is transported in the blood to target tissues- It directly interacts with and activates adrenoreceptors	It is synthesized into the nerve ending

9	10
Ephedrine	Interaction with adrenoreceptors

1

Catecholamine includes

2

Epinephrine decreases intracellular camp levels by acting on

3

True or False. Skeletal muscle vessels have predominantly alfa receptors and constrict in the presence of epinephrine and norepinephrine

4

True or False. ALFA receptors increase arterial resistence, whereas beta2 receptor promote smooth muscle relaxation

5

True or False. The skin and splanchic vessels have predominantly alfa receptors.

6

True or False. Vessels in a skeletal muscle may constrict or dilate depending on whether alfa or beta2 receptors are activated

7

Direct effects on the heart are determined largely by

8

Which of the following effects is related to direct beta1 adrenoreceptor stimulation?

9

Distribution of alfa adrenoreceptor subtypes is associated with all of the following tissues

10

Distribution of alfa adrenoreceptor subtypes is not associated with the tissues of

1 - Epinephrine- Isoprenaline- Norepinephrine	2 α2 receptor
3 FALSE	4 TRUE
5 TRUE	6 TRUE
7 Beta1 receptor	8 Tachycardia
9 - Blood vessels- Prostate- Pupillary dilator muscle	10 HEART

1 Beta adrenoreceptor subtypes is not contained in tissues of	2 Beta adrenoreceptor subtypes is contained in
3 In which tissues both alfa and beta1 adrenergic stimulation produces the same effect?	4 The effects of sympathomimetics on blood pressure are associated with their effects on
5 A relatively pure alfa agonist causes	6 A relatively pure alfa agonist do not causes
7 A nonselective beta receptor agonist causes	8 A nonselective beta receptor agonist do not causes
9 True or False. Alfa agonists cause miosis.	10 True or False. Alfa agonists cause mydriasis.

1	2
Pupillary dilator muscle	- Bronchial muscles- Heart- Fat cells
3	4
Intestine	- The heart- The peripheral resistance- The venous return
5	6
- Increase peripheral arterial resistance- Increase venous return- Reflex bradycardia	Effect on blood vessels
7	8
- Increase cardiac output- Decrease peripheral arterial resistance- Decrease the mean pressure	Increase peripheral arterial resistance
9	10
FALSE	TRUE

1. True or False. Beta antagonists decrease the production of aqueous humor

2. True or False. Alfa agonists increase the outflow of aqueous humor from the eye

3. A bronchial smooth muscle contains

4. All of the following agents are beta receptor agonists

5. All of the following agents are beta receptor agonists EXCEPT

6. Which of the following drugs causes bronchodilation without significant cardiac stimulation?

7. Alfa-receptor stimulation includes

8. Alfa-receptor stimulation do not includes

9. Beta1 receptor stimulation includes

10. Beta1 receptor stimulation do not includes

1	2
TRUE	TRUE

3	4
Beta 2 receptor	- Epinephrine- Isoproterenol- Dobutamine

5	6
Methoxamine	Terbutaline

7	8
- Relaxation of gastrointestinal smooth muscle- Contraction of bladder base, uterus and prostate- Stimulation of platelet aggregation	Stimulation of insulin secretion

9	10
- Increase in contractility- Tachycardia- Increase in conduction velocity in the atrioventricular node	Bronchodilation

1. Beta2 receptor stimulation includes

2. Beta2 receptor stimulation do not includes

3. Hyperglycemia induced by epinephrine is due to

4. Which of the following effects is associated with beta3-receptor stimulation?

5. True or False. Norepinephrine has a predominantly beta action

6. True or False. Epinephrine acts on both alfa- and beta-receptors

7. True or False. Methoxamine has a predominantly alfa action

8. True or False. Isoprenaline has a predominantly beta action

9. Indicate the drug, which is a direct-acting both alfa- and beta-receptor agonist

10. Which of the following agents is an alfa1 alfa2 beta1 beta2 receptor agonist?

1. - Stimulation of renin secretion- Fall of potassium concentration in plasma- Relaxation of bladder, uterus	2. Tachycardia
3. - Gluconeogenesis (beta2)- Inhibition of insulin secretion (alfa)- Stimulation of glycogenolysis (beta2)	4. Lipolysis
5. FALSE	6. TRUE
7. TRUE	8. TRUE
9. Norepinephrine	10. Epinephrine

1

Indicate the direct-acting sympathomimetic, which is an alfa1 alfa2 beta1 receptor agonist

2

Which of the following agents is an alfa1-selective agonist?

3

Indicate the alfa2-selective agonist

4

Which agents is a nonselective beta receptor agonist?

5

Indicate the beta1-selective agonist

6

Which sympathomimetics is a beta2-selective agonist?

7

Indicate the indirect-acting sympathomimetic agent

8

Epinephrine produces all of the following effects

9

Epinephrine produces all of the following effects EXCEPT

10

Epinephrine produces all of the following effects

1 Norepinephrine	2 Methoxamine
3 Xylometazoline	4 Isoproterenol
5 Dobutamine	6 Terbutaline
7 Ephedrine	8 - Positive inotropic and chronotropic actions on the heart (beta1 receptor)- Increase peripheral resistance (alfa receptor)- Skeletal muscle blood vessel dilatation (beta2 receptor)
9 Predominance of alfa effects at low concentration	10 - Bronchodilation- Hyperglycemia- Mydriasis

1. Epinephrine produces all of the following effects EXCEPT

2. Epinephrine is used in the treatment of

3. Epinephrine is not used in the treatment of

4. Compared with epinephrine, norepinephrine do not produces

5. Norepinephrine produces

6. Which direct-acting drugs is a relatively pure alfa agonist, an effective mydriatic and decongestant and can be used to raise blood pressure?

7. Characteristics of methoxamine include

8. Characteristics of methoxamine do not

9. Which agents is an alfa2-selective agonist with ability to promote constriction of the nasal mucosa?

10. Indicate the sympathomimetic, which may cause hypotension, presumably because of a clonidine-like effect

1	2
Decrease in oxygen consumption	- Bronchospasm- Anaphylactic shock- Open-angle glaucoma
3	4
Cardiac arrhythmias	Decrease the mean pressure below normal before returning to the control value
5	6
Vasoconstriction	Phenylephrine
7	8
- It is a direct-acting alfa1-receptor agonist- It causes reflex bradycardia- It increases total peripheral resistance	It increases heart rate, contractility and cardiac output
9	10
Xylometazoline	Xylometazoline

1 Isoproterenol is	2 Isoproterenol produces
3 Isoproterenol do not produces	4 Characteristics of dobutamine is not
5 Characteristics of dobutamine include	6 Characteristics of salmeterol include
7 Characteristics of salmeterol do not include	8 Characteristics of ephedrine include
9 Characteristics of ephedrine do not include	10 Ephedrine causes

1 Nonselective beta receptor agonist	2 - Increase in cardiac output- Fall in diastolic and mean arterial pressure- Tachycardia
3 Bronchoconstriction	4 It is used to treat bronchospasm
5 - It is a relatively beta1-selective synthetic catecholamine- It increases atrioventricular conduction- It causes minimal changes in heart rate and systolic pressure	6 - It is a potent selective beta2 agonist- It causes uterine relaxation- It is used in the therapy of asthma
7 It stimulates heart rate, contractility and cardiac output	8 - It acts primarily through the release of stored cathecholamines- It is a mild CNS stimulant- It causes tachyphylaxis with repeated administration
9 It decreases arterial pressure	10 Bronchodilation

1	2
Compared with epinephrine, ephedrine produces	Compared with epinephrine, ephedrine do not produces
3	4
Which sympathomimetics is preferable for the treatment of chronic orthostatic hypotension?	Indicate the sympathomimetic drug, which is used in a hypotensive emergency
5	6
Which sympathomimetics is preferable for the emergency therapy of cardiogenic shock?	Indicate the sympathomimetic agent, which is combined with a local anesthetic to prolong the duration of infiltration nerve block
7	8
Which sympathomimetics is related to short-acting topical decongestant agents?	Indicate the long-acting topical decongestant agents
9	10
Which topical decongestant agents is an alfa2-selective agonist?	Indicate the sympathomimetic, which may be useful in the emergency management of cardiac arrest

1	2
- It has oral activity- It is resistant to MAO and has much longer duration of action- Its effects are similar, but it is less potent	It is a direct-acting sympathomimetic
3	4
Ephedrine	Phenylephrine
5	6
Dobutamine	Epinephrine
7	8
Phenylephrine	Xylometazoline
9	10
Xylometazoline	Epinephrine

1. Which sympathomimetics is used in the therapy of bronchial asthma?

2. Indicate the agent of choice in the emergency therapy of anaphylactic shock

3. Which sympathomimetics is an effective mydriatic?

4. The adverse effects of sympathomimetics include

5. The adverse effects of sympathomimetics do not include

6. Which drugs is a nonselective alfa receptor antagonist?

7. Indicate the alfa1-selective antagonist

8. Which agents is an alfa2–selective antagonist?

9. Indicate the irreversible alfa receptor antagonist

10. Which drugs is an nonselective beta receptor antagonist?

1	2
Formoterol	Epinephrine

3	4
Phenylephrine	- Cerebral hemorrhage or pulmonary edema - Myocardial infarction - Ventricular arrhythmias

5	6
Drug-induced parkinsonism	Phentolamine

7	8
Prazosin	Yohimbine

9	10
Phenoxybenzamine	Propranolol

1. Indicate the beta1-selective antagonist

2. Which of the following agents is a beta2–selective antagonist?

3. Indicate the beta adrenoreceptor antagonist, which has partial beta–agonist activity

4. Which drugs is a reversible nonselective alfa, beta antagonist?

5. Indicate the indirect-acting adrenoreceptor blocking drug

6. The principal mechanism of action of adrenoreceptor antagonists is

7. Characteristics of alfa-receptor antagonists do not include

8. Which drugs is an imidazoline derivative and a potent competitive antagonist at both alfa1 and alfa2 receptors?

9. Characteristics of phentolamine include

10. Characteristics of phentolamine do not include

1	2
Metoprolol	Butoxamine
3	4
Pindolol	Labetalol
5	6
Reserpine	Reversible or irreversible interaction with adrenoreceptors
7	8
Bronchospasm	Phentolamine
9	10
- Reduction in peripheral resistance- Tachycardia- Stimulation of muscarinic, H1 and H2 histamine receptors	Stimulation of responses to serotonin

1. The principal mechanism of phentolamine-induced tachycardia is

2. Nonselective alfa-receptor antagonists are most useful in the treatment of

3. The main reason for using alfa-receptor antagonists in the management of pheochromocytoma is

4. Which drugs is useful in the treatment of pheochromocytoma?

5. Indicate adrenoreceptor antagonist agents, which are used for the management of pheochromocytoma

6. The principal adverse effects of phentolamine include

7. The principal adverse effects of phentolamine do not include

8. Indicate the reversible nonselective alfa-receptor antagonist, which is an ergot derivative

9. Indicate an alfa-receptor antagonist, which binds covalently to alfa receptors, causing irreversible blockade of long duration (14-48 hours or longer)

10. Compared with phentolamine, prazosin has all of the following features

1 Antagonism of presynaptic alfa2 receptors enhances norepinephrine release, which causes cardiac stimulation via unblocked beta receptors	**2** Pheochromocytoma
3 Blockade of alfa2 receptors on vascular smooth muscle results in epinephrine stimulation of unblocked alfa2 receptors	**4** Phentolamine
5 Alfa-receptor antagonists	**6** - Diarrhea - Arrhythmias - Myocardial ischemia
7 Bradycardia	**8** Ergotamine
9 Phenoxybenzamine	**10** - Highly selective for alfa1 receptors - The relative absence of tachycardia - Persistent block of alfa1 receptors

1. Compared with phentolamine, prazosin has not features

2. True or False. ALFA1a subtype mediates both vascular and prostate smooth muscle contraction

3. True or False. There are at least three subtypes of alfa1 receptors, designated alfa1a, alfa1b and alfa1d

4. True or False. ALFA1a subtype mediates prostate smooth muscle contraction

5. True or False. ALFA1b subtype mediates vascular smooth muscle contraction

6. Indicate an alfa1 adrenoreceptor antagonist, which has great selectivity for alfa1a subtype

7. Subtype-selective alfa1 receptor antagonists such as tamsulosin, terazosin, alfusosin are efficacious in

8. Indicate an alfa receptor antagonist, which is an efficacious drug in the treatment of mild to moderate systemic hypertension

9. Beta-blocking drugs-induced chronically lower blood pressure may be associated with theirs effects on

10. Characteristics of beta-blocking agents do not include

1 Irreversible blockade of alfa receptors	2 FALSE
3 TRUE	4 TRUE
5 TRUE	6 Tamsulosin
7 Benign prostatic hyperplasia (BPH)	8 Prazosin
9 - The heart- The blood vessels- The renin-angiotensin system	10 They induce depression and depleted stores of catecholamines

1	2
Beta-receptor antagonists have all of the following cardiovascular effects	Beta-receptor antagonists have not the following cardiovascular effects
3	**4**
Beta-blocking agents have all of the following effects	Beta-blocking agents have all of the following effects except
5	**6**
Beta-receptor antagonists cause	Propranolol has all of the following cardiovascular effects
7	**8**
Propranolol has all of the following cardiovascular effects except	Propranolol-induced adverse effects include
9	**10**
Propranolol-induced adverse effects do not include	Propranolol is used in the treatment all of the following diseases

1 - The negative inotropic and chronotropic effects- Vasoconstriction- Reduction of the release of renin	**2** Acute effects of these drugs include a fall in peripheral resistance
3 - Bronchoconstriction- Decrease of aqueous humor prodaction- "membrane-stabilizing" action	**4** Increase plasma concentrations of HDL and decrease of VLDL
5 Inhibition of glycogenolysis	**6** - It decreases cardiac work and oxygen demand- It inhibits the renin secretion- It increases the atrioventricular nodal refractory period
7 It reduces blood flow to the brain	**8** - Bronchoconstriction- "supersensitivity" of beta-adrenergic receptors (rapid withdrawal)- Sedation, sleep disturbances, depression and sexual dysfunction
9 Hyperglycemia	**10** - Cardiovascular diseases- Hyperthyroidism- Migraine headache

1. Propranolol is used in the treatment all of the following diseases except

2. Metoprolol and atenolol are members of

3. Which beta receptor antagonists is preferable in patients with asthma, diabetes or peripheral vascular diseases?

4. Indicate a beta receptor antagonist, which has very long duration of action

5. Indicate a beta1-selective receptor antagonist, which has very long duration of action

6. Which drugs is a nonselective beta-blocker without intrinsic sympathomimetic or local anesthetic activity and used for the treatment of life-threatening ventricular arrhythmias?

7. Indicate a beta receptor antagonist with intrinsic sympathomimetic activity

8. Pindolol, oxprenolol have all of the following properties

9. Which drugs has both alfa1-selective and beta-blocking effects?

10. Characteristics of carvedilol include

1 Bronchial asthma	2 The beta1-selective group
3 Metoprolol	4 Nadolol
5 Betaxolol	6 Sotalol
7 Oxprenolol	8 - They are nonselective beta antagonists- They are less likely to cause bradycardia and abnormalities in plasma lipids- They are effective in hypertension and angina
9 Labetalol	10 - It has both alfa1-selective and beta-blocking effects- It attenuates oxygen free radical-initiated lipid peroxidation- It inhibits vascular smooth muscle mitogenesis

1. Characteristics of carvedilol do not include	2. Indicate the adrenoreceptor antagonist drug, which is a rauwolfia alkaloid
3. Characteristics of reserpine do not include	4. Indicate a beta-blocker, which is particularly efficacious in thyroid storm
5. Beta-receptor blocking drugs are used in the treatment all of the following diseases	6. Beta-receptor blocking drugs are used in the treatment all of the following diseases except
7. Beta-blocker-induced adverse effects include	8. Beta-blocker-induced adverse effects do not include
9. Hypnotic drugs are used to treat	10. Hypnotic drugs should

1 It is a beta1-selective antagonist	2 Reserpine
3 It inhibits the uptake of norepinephrine into vesicles and MAO	4 Propranolol
5 - Hypertension, ischemic heart disease, cardiac arrhythmias- Glaucoma- Hyperthyroidism	6 Pheochromocytoma
7 - Bronchoconstriction- Depression of myocardial contractility and excitability- "supersensitivity" of beta-receptors associated with rapid withdrawal of drugs	8 Hyperglycemia
9 Sleep disorders	10 Produce drowsiness, encourage the onset and maintenance of sleep

1. Which chemical agents are used in the treatment of insomnia?

2. Select a hypnotic drug, which is a benzodiazepine derivative

3. Tick a hypnotic agent – a barbituric acid derivative

4. Select a hypnotic drug, which is an imidazopyridine derivative

5. Which hypnotic agents is absorbed slowly?

6. Which barbiturates is an ultra-short-acting drug?

7. Indicate the barbituric acid derivative, which has 4-5 days elimination half-life

8. Indicate the hypnotic benzodiazepine, which has the shortest elimination half-life

9. Which hypnotic drugs is more likely to cause cumulative and residual effects?

10. Which hypnotic drugs increases the activity of hepatic drug-metabolizing enzyme systems?

1 - Benzodiazepines- Imidazopyridines- Barbiturates	2 Flurazepam
3 Thyopental	4 Zolpidem
5 Temazepam	6 Thiopental
7 Phenobarbital	8 Triazolam
9 Phenobarbital	10 Phenobarbital

1. Hepatic microsomal drug-metabolizing enzyme induction leads to

2. True or False. Hypnotic benzodiazepines are more powerful enzyme inducers than barbiturates.

3. Indicate the hypnotic drug, which does not change hepatic drug-metabolizing enzyme activity?

4. Barbiturates increase the rate of metabolism of

5. Which agents inhibits hepatic metabolism of hypnotics?

6. Which factors can influence the biodisposition of hypnotic agents?

7. Which hypnotics is preferred for elderly patients?

8. Which hypnotics is preferred in patients with limited hepatic function?

9. Indicate the mechanism of barbiturate action (at hypnotic doses)

10. Imidazopyridines are

1 Barbiturate tolerance	2 FALSE
3 - Flurazepam- Zaleplon- Triazolam	4 - Anticoagulants- Digitalis compounds- Glucocorticoids
5 Cimetidin	6 - Alterations in the hepatic function resulting from a disease- Old age- Drug-induced increases or decreases in microsomal enzyme activities
7 Temazepam	8 Zolpidem
9 Increasing the duration of the GABA-gated Cl- channel openings	10 Selective agonists of the BZ1 (omega1) subtype of BZ receptors

1. Which hypnotic agents is a positive allosteric modulator of GABA-A receptor function?

2. Indicate a hypnotic drug - a selective agonist at the BZ1 receptor subtype

3. Which hypnotic agents is able to interact with both BZ1 and BZ2 receptor subtypes?

4. Indicate the competitive antagonist of BZ receptors

5. Flumazenil blocks the actions of

6. Indicate the agent, which interferes with GABA binding

7. Which agents blocks the chloride channel directly?

8. Which agents is preferred in the treatment of insomnia?

9. Barbiturates are being replaced by hypnotic benzodiazepines because of

10. Which benzodiazepines is used mainly for hypnosis?

1	2
- Zaleplon - Flurazepam - Zolpidem	Zolpidem
3	4
Flurazepam	Flumazenil
5	6
Zolpidem	Bicuculline
7	8
Picrotoxin	Hypnotic benzodiazepines
9	10
- Low therapeutic index - Suppression in REM sleep - High potential of physical dependence and abuse	Flurazepam

1 Indicate the main claim for an ideal hypnotic agent

2 Which stage of sleep is responsible for the incidence of dreams?

3 During slow wave sleep (stage 3 and 4 NREM sleep)

4 All of the hypnotic drugs induce

5 Which hypnotic drugs causes least suppression of REM sleep?

6 Although the benzodiazepines continue to be the agents of choice for insomnia, they have

7 Hypnotic benzodiazepines can cause

8 Which hypnotic benzodiazepines is more likely to cause rebound insomnia?

9 Which hypnotic benzodiazepines is more likely to cause "hangover" effects such as drowsiness, dysphoria, and mental or motor depression the following day?

10 Indicate the hypnotic drug, which binds selectively to the BZ1 receptor subtype, facilitating GABAergic inhibition

1	2
- Rapid onset and sufficient duration of action - Minor effects on sleep patterns - Minimal "hangover" effects	REM sleep

3	4
Somnambulism and nightmares occur	Decrease the duration of REM sleep

5	6
Flurazepam	- The possibility of psychological and physiological dependence - Synergistic depression of CNS with other drugs (especially alcohol) - Residual drowsiness and daytime sedation

7	8
A dose-dependent decrease in both REM and slow wave sleep	Triazolam

9	10
Flurazepam	Zolpidem

1. Which agent exerts hypnotic activity with minimal muscle relaxing and anticonvulsant effects?

2. True or False. Zolpidem and zaleplon have effectiveness similar to that of hypnotic benzodiazepines in the management of sleep disorders.

3. Which hypnotic drugs is used intravenously as anesthesia?

4. Indicate the usual cause of death due to overdose of hypnotics

5. Toxic doses of hypnotics may cause a circulatory collapse as a result of

6. The mechanism of action of antiseizure drugs is

7. Which antiseizure drugs produces enhancement of GABA-mediated inhibition?

8. Indicate an antiseizure drug, which has an impotent effect on the T-type calcium channels in thalamic neurons?

9. Which antiseizure drugs produces a voltage-dependent inactivation of sodium channels?

10. Indicate an antiseizure drug, inhibiting central effects of excitatory amino acids

1 Zaleplon	2 TRUE
3 Thiopental	4 Depression of the medullar respiratory center
5 Action on the medullar vasomotor center	6 - Enhancement of GABAergic (inhibitory) transmission - Diminution of excitatory (usually glutamatergic) transmission - Modification of ionic conductance
7 Phenobarbital	8 Ethosuximide
9 - Lamotrigine - Carbamazepin - Phenytoin	10 Lamotrigine

1 The drug for partial and generalized tonic-clonic seizures is	2 Indicate an anti-absence drug
3 The drug against myoclonic seizures is	4 The most effective drug for stopping generalized tonic-clonic status epilepticus in adults is
5 Phenytoin	6 Phenytoin is used in the treatment of
7 Dose-related adverse effect caused by phenytoin is	8 Granulocytopenia, gastrointestinal irritation, gingival hyperplasia, and facial hirsutism are possible adverse effects of
9 The antiseizure drug, which induces hepatic microsomal enzymes, is	10 The drug of choice for partial seizures is

1	2
- Carbamazepine- Valproate- Phenytoin	Valproate

3	4
Clonazepam	Diazepam

5	6
It blocks sodium channels	Grand mal epilepsy

7	8
Gingival hyperplasia	Phenytoin

9	10
Phenytoin	Carbamazepin

1 The mechanism of action of carbamazepine appears to be similar to that of	**2** Which antiseizure drugs is also effective in treating trigeminal neuralgia?
3 The most common dose-related adverse effects of carbamazepine are	**4** Indicate the drug of choice for status epilepticus in infants and children
5 Barbiturates are used in the emergency treatment of status epilepticus in infants and children because of	**6** Which antiseizure drugs binds to an allosteric regulatory site on the GABA-BZ receptor, increases the duration of the Cl-channels openings
7 Adverse effect caused by phenobarbital is	**8** Which antiseizure drugs is a prodrug, metabolized to phenobarbital?
9 Indicate the antiseizure drug, which is a phenyltriazine derivative	**10** Lamotrigine can be used in the treatment of

1	2
Phenytoin	Carbamazepine

3	4
Diplopia, ataxia, and nausea	Phenobarbital sodium

5	6
They significantly decrease of oxygen utilization by the brain, protecting cerebral edema and ischemia	Phenobarbital

7	8
- Physical and phychological dependence- Exacerbated petit mal epilepsy- Sedation	Primidone

9	10
Lamotrigine	- Partial seizures- Absence- Myoclonic seizures

1 The mechanism of vigabatrin's action is	2 Indicate an irreversible inhibitor of GABA aminotransferase (GABA-T)
3 Tiagabine	4 The mechanism of both topiramate and felbamate action is
5 The drug of choice in the treatment of petit mal (absence seizures) is	6 The dose-related adverse effect of ethosuximide is
7 Valproate is very effective against	8 The drug of choice in the treatment of myoclonic seizures is
9 The reason for preferring ethosuximide to valproate for uncomplicated absence seizures is	10 Indicate the antiseizure drug, which is a sulfonamide derivative, blocking Na+ channels and having additional ability to inhibit T-type Ca2+ channels

1	2
Inhibition of GABA aminotransferase	Vigabatrin
3	4
Blocks neuronal and glial reuptake of GABA from synapses	- Reduction of excitatory glutamatergic neurotransmission- Inhibition of voltage sensitive Na+ channels- Potentiation of GABAergic neuronal transmission
5	6
Ethosuximide	- Gastrointestinal reactions, such as anorexia, pain, nausea and vomiting- Exacerbated grand mal epilepsy- Transient lethargy or fatigue
7	8
- Absence seizures- Myoclonic seizures- Generalized tonic-clonic seizures	Valproate
9	10
Valproate's idiosyncratic hepatotoxicity	Zonisamide

1. Indicate the antiseizure drug – a benzodiazepine receptor agonist

2. Which antiseizure drugs acts directly on the GABA receptor-chloride channel complex?

3. Benzodiazepine's uselfulness is limited by

4. A long-acting drug against both absence and myoclonic seizures is

5. Which antiseizure drugs may produce teratogenicity?

6. The most dangerous effect of antiseizure drugs after large overdoses is

7. Which neurons are involved in parkinsonism?

8. The pathophysiologic basis for antiparkinsonism therapy is

9. Which neurotransmitters is involved in Parkinson's disease?

10. True or False. The concentration of dopamine in the basal ganglia of the brain is reduced in parkinsonism.

1	2
Lorazepam	Diazepam

3	4
Tolerance	Clonazepam

5	6
- Phenytoin- Valproate- Topiramate	Respiratory depression

7	8
- Cholinergic neurons- GABAergic neurons- Dopaminergic neurons	A selective loss of dopaminergic neurons

9	10
- Acetylcholine- Glutamate- Dopamine	TRUE

1. Indicate the drug that induces parkinsonian syndromes

2. Which drugs is used in the treatment of Parkinsonian disorders

3. Select the agent, which is preferred in the treatment of the drug-induced form of parkinsonism

4. Which agents is the precursor of dopamine?

5. The main reason for giving levodopa, the precursor of dopamine, instead of dopamine is

6. Indicate a peripheral dopa decarboxylase inhibitor

7. The mechanism of carbidopa's action is

8. True or False. Carbidopa is unable to penetrate the blood-brain barrier, it acts to reduce the peripheral conversion of levodopa to dopamine.

9. Which preparations combines carbidopa and levodopa in a fixed proportion?

10. Gastrointestinal irritation, cardiovascular effects, including tachycardia, arrhythmias, and orthostatic hypotension, mental disturbances, and withdrawal are possible adverse effects of

1 Chlorpromazine	2 Selegiline
3 Benztropine	4 Levodopa
5 Dopamine does not cross the blood-brain barrier	6 Carbidopa
7 Inhibition of dopa decarboxilase	8 TRUE
9 Sinemet	10 Levodopa

1. Which agents is the most helpful in counteracting the behavioral complications of levodopa?

2. Which vitamins reduces the beneficial effects of levodopa by enhancing its extracerebral metabolism?

3. Which drugs antagonizes the effects of levodopa because it leads to a junctional blockade of dopamine action?

4. Levodopa should not be given to patients taking

5. Indicate D2 receptor agonist with antiparkinsonian activity

6. Which antiparkinsonian drugs has also been used to treat hyperprolactinemia?

7. Indicate a selective inhibitor of monoamine oxidase B

8. True or False. MAO-A metabolizes norepinephrine and serotonin, MAO-B metabolizes dopamine

9. True or False. Treatment with selegilin postpones the need for levodopa for 3-9 months and may retard the progression of Parkinson's disease.

10. The main reason for avoiding the combined administration of levodopa and an inhibitor of both forms of monoamine oxidase is

1 Clozapine	2 Pyridoxine
3 - Reserpine- Haloperidol- Chlorpromazine	4 Monoamine oxydase A inhibitors
5 Bromocriptine	6 Bromocriptine
7 Selegiline	8 TRUE
9 TRUE	10 Hypertensive emergency

1. Indicate selective catechol-O-methyltransferase inhibitor, which prolongs the action of levodopa by diminishing its peripheral metabolism

2. Which antiparkinsonian drugs is an antiviral agent used in the prophylaxis of influenza A2?

3. The mechanism of amantadine action is

4. Which antiparkinsonism drugs is an anticholinergic agent?

5. Mental confusion and hallucinations, peripheral atropine like toxicity (e.g. Cycloplegia, tachycardia, urinary retention, and constipation) are possible adverse effects of

6. Indicate the antiparkinsonism drug which should be avoided in patients with glaucoma

7. Alcohol may cause

8. Alcohol

9. True or False. It is undesirable to take alcohol before going outdoors when it extremely cold, but it may be harmless to take some after coming into a warm place from the cold.

10. The most common medical complication of alcohol abuse is

1 Tolcapone	2 Amantadine
3 Stimulating the glutamatergic neurotransmission	4 Trihexyphenidyl
5 Benztropine	6 Trihexyphenidyl
7 - CNS depression- Vasodilatation- Hypoglycemia	8 Increases body heat loss
9 TRUE	10 - Liver failure including liver cirrhosis- Tolerance and physical dependence- Generalized symmetric peripheral nerve injury, ataxia and dementia

1	2
Effect of moderate consumption of alcohol on plasma lipoproteins is	Which metabolic alterations may be associated with chronic alcohol abuse?
3	4
Alcohol potentiates	Which drugs is most commonly used for causing a noxious reaction to alcohol by blocking its metabolism?
5	6
Which agents is an inhibitor of aldehyde dehydrogenase?	Indicate the drug, which alters brain responses to alcohol
7	8
Which agents is an opioid antagonist?	Alcohol causes an acute increase in the local concentrations of
9	10
Management of alcohol withdrawal syndrome contains	Indicate the drug, which decreases the craving for alcohol or blunts pleasurable "high" that comes with renewed drinking

1 Raising serum levels of high-density lipoproteins	2 Severe loss of potassium and magnesium
3 - SNS depressants- Vasodilatators- Hypoglycemic agents	4 Disulfiram
5 Disulfiram	6 Naltrexone
7 Naltrexone	8 - Dopamine- Opioid- Serotonine
9 - Restoration of potassium, magnesium and phosphate balance- Thiamine therapy- Substituting a long-acting sedative-hypnotic drug for alcohol	10 Naltrexone

1 The symptoms resulting from the combination of disulfiram and alcohol are	**2** The combination of disulfiram and ethanol leads to accumulation of
3 True or False. The combination of naltrexone and disulfiram should be avoided since both drugs are potential hepatotoxins.	**4** Indicate the "specific" modality of treatment for severe methanol poisoning
5 Which agents may be used as an antidote for ethylene glycol and methanol poisoning?	**6** The principal mechanism of fomepizol action is associated with inhibition of
7 Narcotics analgesics should	**8** Second-order pain is
9 Chemical mediators in the nociceptive pathway are	**10** Chemical mediators in the nociceptive pathway are not

1 Nausea, vomiting	2 Acetaldehyde
3 TRUE	4 - Dialysis to enhance removal of methanol- Alkalinization to counteract metabolic acidosis- Suppression of metabolism by alcohol dehydrogenase to toxic products
5 Fomepizol	6 Alcohol dehydrogenase
7 Relieve severe pain	8 Dull, burning pain
9 - Kinins- Prostaglandins- Substance P	10 Enkephalins

1 Indicate the chemical mediator in the antinociceptive descending pathways	**2** Which mediators is found mainly in long descending pathways from the midbrain to the dorsal horn?
3 Select the brain and spinal cord regions, which are involved in the transmission of pain?	**4** Mu (μ) receptors are associated with
5 Which opioid receptor types is responsible for euphoria and respiratory depression?	**6** Indicate the opioid receptor type, which is responsible for dysphoria and vasomotor stimulation
7 Kappa and delta agonists	**8** Which supraspinal structures is implicated in pain-modulating descending pathways?
9 Indicate the neurons, which are located in the locus ceruleus or the lateral tegmental area of the reticular formation	**10** Which analgesics is a phenanthrene derivative?

1 - BETA-endorphin- Met- and leu-enkephalin- Dynorphin	2 Enkephalin
3 - The limbic system, including the amygdaloidal nucleus and the hypothalamus- The ventral and medial parts of the thalamus- The substantia gelatinosa	4 Analgesia, euphoria, respiratory depression, physical dependence
5 Mu (μ) receptors	6 Kappa-receptors
7 Close a voltage-gated Ca2+ channels on presynaptic nerve terminals	8 The midbrain periaqueductal gray
9 Nonadrenergic	10 Morphine

1

Tick narcotic analgesic, which is a phenylpiperidine derivative

2

Which opioid analgesics is a strong mu receptor agonist?

3

Indicate the narcotic analgesic, which is a natural agonist

4

Select the narcotic analgesic, which is an antagonist or partial mu receptor agonist

5

Which agents is a full antagonist of opioid receptors?

6

The principal central nervous system effect of the opioid analgesics with affinity for a mu receptor is

7

Which opioid analgesics can produce dysphoria, anxiety and hallucinations?

8

Which opioid analgesics is used in combination with droperidol in neuroleptanalgesia?

9

Fentanyl can produce significant respiratory depression by

10

Most strong mu receptor agonists cause

1 Fentanyl	2 Morphine
3 Morphine	4 Pentazocine
5 Naloxone	6 - Analgesia- Respiratory depression- Euphoria
7 Pentazocine	8 Fentanyl
9 - Suppression of the cough reflex leading to airway obstruction- Development of truncal rigidity	10 Cerebral vasodilatation, causing an increase in intracranial pressure

1	2
Which opioid analgesics can produce an increase in the pulmonary arterial pressure and myocardial work?	Morphine causes

3	4
Morphine do not causes	Therapeutic doses of the opioid analgesics

5	6
Which opioid analgesics is used in obstetric labor?	Indicate the opioid analgesic, which is used for relieving the acute, severe pain of renal colic

7	8
Which opioid analgesics is used in the treatment of acute pulmonary edema?	The relief produced by intravenous morphine in dyspnea from pulmonary edema is associated with reduced

9	10
Rhinorrhea, lacrimation, chills, gooseflesh, hyperventilation, hyperthermia, mydriasis, muscular aches, vomiting, diarrhea, anxiety, and hostility are effects of	The diagnostic triad of opioid overdosage is

1	2
Pentazocine	- Constipation- Urinary retention- Bronchiolar constriction
3	4
Dilatation of the biliary duct	Decrease body temperature
5	6
Meperidine	Meperidine
7	8
Morphine	- Perception of shortness of breath- Patient anxiety- Cardiac preload (reduced venous tone) and afterload (decreased peripheral resistance)
9	10
Abstinence syndrome	Coma, depressed respiration and miosis

1. Which opioid agents is used in the treatment of acute opioid overdose?

2. Indicate the pure opioid antagonist, which has a half-life of 10 hours

3. In contrast to morphine, methadone

4. Which opioid analgesics is a partial mu receptor agonist?

5. Indicate a partial mu receptor agonist, which has 20-60 times analgesic potency of morphine, and a longer duration of action

6. Which opioid analgesics is a strong kappa receptor agonist and a mu receptor antagonist?

7. Which drugs has weak mu agonist effects and inhibitory action on norepinephrine and serotonin reuptake in the CNS?

8. Non-narcotic analgesics are mainly effective against pain associated with

9. Non-narcotic agents cause

10. Non-narcotic analgesics are

1	2
Naloxone	Naltrexone

3	4
- Causes tolerance and physical dependence more slowly- Is more effective orally- Withdrawal is less severe, although more prolonged	Buprenorphine

5	6
Buprenorphine	Nalbuphine

7	8
Tramadol	Inflammation or tissue damage

9	10
Antipyretic effect	- Paracetamol- Acetylsalicylic acid- Ketorolac

1. Non-narcotic analgesics are not

2. Select the non-narcotic drug, which is a paraaminophenol derivative

3. Which of the following non-narcotic agents is salicylic acid derivative?

4. Tick pirazolone derivative

5. Which non-narcotic agents inhibits mainly cyclooxygenase (COX) in CNS?

6. Most of non-narcotic analgetics have

7. Indicate the non-narcotic analgesic, which lacks an anti-inflammatory effect

8. True or False about aspirin. It inhibits mainly peripheral COX

9. True or False about aspirin. It does not have an anti-inflammatory effect

10. True or False about aspirin. It inhibits platelet aggregation.

1	2
Butorphanol	Paracetamol
3	4
Aspirin	Analgin
5	6
Paracetamol	- Anti-inflammatory effect- Analgesic effect- Antipyretic effect
7	8
Paracetamol	TRUE
9	10
FALSE	TRUE

1 True or False about aspirin. It stimulates respiration by a direct action on the respiratory center	**2** For which conditions could aspirin be used prophylactically?
3 All of the following are undesirable effects of aspirin	**4** Is not a Undesirable effects of aspirin
5 Characteristic findinds of salicylism include	**6** Analgin usefulness is limited by
7 Methemoglobinemia is possible adverse effect of	**8** True or False for ketorolac. It inhibits COX
9 True or False for ketorolac. It is as effective as morphine for a short-term relief from moderate to severe pain	**10** True or False for ketorolac. It has a high potential for physical dependence and abuse

1 TRUE	2 Thromboembolism
3 - Gastritis with focal erosions- Bleeding due to a decrease of platelet aggregation- Reversible renal insufficiency	4 Tolerance and physical addiction
5 - Headache, mental confusion and drowsiness- Tinnitus and difficulty in hearing- Hyperthermia, sweating, thirst, hyperventilation, vomiting and diarrhea	6 Agranulocytosis
7 Paracetamol	8 TRUE
9 TRUE	10 FALSE

1. True or False for ketorolac. It does not produce respiratory depression

2. Indicate the nonopioid agent of central effect with analgesic activity

3. Select the antiseizure drug with an analgesic component of effect

4. Which nonopioid agents is an antidepressant with analgesic activity?

5. Tick mixed (opioid/non-opioid) agent

6. Neuroleptics are used to treat

7. Most antipsychotic drugs

8. Which dopaminergic systems is most closely related to behavior?

9. Hyperprolactinemia is caused by blockade of dopamine in

10. Parkinsonian symptoms and tarditive dyskinesia are caused by blockade dopamine in

1	2
TRUE	Clopheline
3	4
Carbamazepine	Amitriptyline
5	6
Tramadol	Psychosis
7	8
Strongly block postsynaptic d2receptor	The mesolimbic and mesofrontal systems
9	10
The pituitary	The nigrostriatal system

1

Extrapyramidal reactions can be treated by

2

True or False. D1 postsynaptic receptors are located in striatum

3

True or False. D2 pre- and postsynaptic receptors are located in striatum and limbic areas

4

True or False. D4 postsynaptic receptors are located in frontal cortex, mesolimbic system

5

Which antipsychotic drugs is typical?

6

Indicate the atypical antipsychotic drug

7

Atypical antipsychotic agents (such as clozapine) differ from typical ones

8

Tardive dyskinesia is the result of

9

Which antipsychotic drugs has high affinity for D4 and 5-HT2 receptors?

10

Indicate the antipsychotic drug, which is a phenothiazine aliphatic derivative

1	2
Benztropine mesylate	TRUE
3	4
TRUE	TRUE
5	6
Haloperidol	Clozapine
7	8
- In reduced risks of extrapyramidal system dysfunction and tardive dyscinesia- In having low affinity for D1 and D2 dopamine receptors- In having high affinity for D4 dopamine receptors	Hyperactive dopaminergic state in the presence of dopamine blockers
9	10
Clozapine	Chlorpromazine

1	2
Indicate the antipsychotic drug, which is a butyrophenone derivative	Indicate the antipsychotic drug, which is a thioxanthene derivative
3	4
Indicate the antipsychotic agent – a dibenzodiazepine derivative	The strong antiemetic effect of the phenothiazine derivatives is due to dopamine receptor blockade
5	6
Phenothiazine derivatives are able to	Most phenothiazine derivatives have
7	8
Indicate the antipsychotic drug having significant peripheral alpha-adrenergic blocking activity	Indicate the antipsychotic drug having a muscarinic-cholinergic blocking activity
9	10
Indicate the antipsychotic drug having H1-antihistaminic activity	Parkinson's syndrome, acute dystonic reactions, tardive dyskinesia, antimuscarinic actions, orthostatic hypotension, galactorrhea are possible adverse effects of

1 Droperidol	2 Thiothixene
3 Clozapine	4 - In the chemoreceptor trigger zone of the medulla- Of the receptors in the stomach- The medullar vomiting centre
5 Alter temperature-regulating mechanisms producing hypothermia	6 - Antihistaminic activity- Anticholinergic activity- Antidopaminergic activity
7 Chlorpromazine	8 Chlorpromazine
9 - Clozapine- Chlorpromazine- Olanzapine	10 Chlorpromazine

1. Orthostatic hypotension can occur as a result of

2. Adverse peripheral effects, such as loss of accommodation, dry mouth, tachycardia, urinary retention, constipation are related to

3. Which phenothiazine derivatives is a potent local anesthetic?

4. Which phenothiazine derivatives may produce cardiac toxicity, including ventricular arrhythmias, cardiac conduction block, and sudden death?

5. Which antipsychotic agents is preferable in patients with coronary and cerebrovascular disease?

6. Which antipsychotic agents is used in combination with an opioid drug fentanyl in neuroleptanalgesia?

7. The mechanism of haloperidol antipsychotic action is

8. True or False about clozapine. Has potent anticholinergic activity

9. True or False about clozapine. Has high affinity for D1 and D2 dopamine receptors

10. True or False about clozapine. Produces significant extrapyramidal toxicity

1 - The central action of phenothiazines- Inhibition of norepinephrine uptake mechanisms- Alpha adrenoreceptor blockade	2 Muscarinic cholinoreceptor blockade
3 Chlorpromazine	4 Thioridazine
5 Haloperidol	6 Droperidol
7 - Blocking D2 receptors- Central alpha-adrenergic blocking- Inhibition of norepinephrine uptake mechanisms	8 TRUE
9 FALSE	10 FALSE

1. True or False about clozapine. Is related to typical antipsychotic agents

2. Which antipsychotic drugs has the high risk of potentially fatal agranulocytosis and risk of seizures at high doses?

3. Which antipsychotic drugs has high affinity for D2 and 5-HT2 receptors?

4. Lithium carbonate is useful in the treatment of

5. The drug of choice for manic-depressive psychosis is

6. The lithium mode of action is

7. True or False about lithium. Stimulate dopamine and beta-adrenergic receptors

8. True or False about lithium. Decrease catecholamine-related activity

9. True or False about lithium. Stimulate the development of dopamine receptor supersensitivity

10. True or False about lithium. Decrease cholinergic activity

1. FALSE	2. Clozapine
3. Risperidone	4. Bipolar disorder
5. Lithium carbonate	6. - Effect on electrolytes and ion transport - Effect on neurotransmitters - Effect on second messengers
7. FALSE	8. TRUE
9. FALSE	10. FALSE

1. Which adverse effects is associated with lithium treatment?

2. The principal mechanism of action of antidepressant agents is

3. Which agents is related to tricyclic antidepressants?

4. Indicate the second-generation heterocyclic drug

5. Which agents is related to the third-generation heterocyclic antidepressants?

6. Which antidepressants is a selective serotonin reuptake inhibitor?

7. Which antidepressant agents is a selective inhibitor of norepinephrine reuptake?

8. Indicate the antidepressant, which blocks the reuptake pumps for serotonin and norepinephrine

9. Which antidepressants is an unselective MAO blocker and produces extremely long-lasting inhibition of the enzyme?

10. Indicate the irreversible MAO inhibitor, which is a hydrazide derivative

1	2
- Cardiovascular anomalies in the newborn- Thyroid enlargement- Nephrogenic diabetes insipidus	Blocking epinephrine or serotonin reuptake pumps
3	4
Amitriptyline	Maprotiline
5	6
Nefazodone	Fluoxetine
7	8
Maprotiline	Amitriptyline
9	10
Tranylcypramine	Phenelzine

1 Which MAO inhibitors has amphetamine-like activity and is related to nonhydrazide derivatives	**2** Which antidepressants is a selective short-acting MAO-A inhibitor?
3 Monoamine Oxydase A	**4** Which synapses are involved in depression?
5 Block of which type of Monoamine Oxydase might be more selective for depression?	**6** The principal mechanism of MAO inhibitor action is
7 The irreversible MAO inhibitors have a very high risk of developing	**8** The most dangerous pharmacodynamic interaction is between MAO inhibitors and
9 Serotonin syndrome is a result of	**10** The therapeutic response to antidepressant drugs is usually over a period of

1 Tranylcypramine	2 Moclobemide
3 Is responsible for norepinephrine, serotonin, and tyramine metabolism	4 Serotoninergic synapses
5 MAO-A	6 Blocking a major degradative pathway for the amine neurotransmitters, which permits more amines to accumulate in presynaptic stores
7 Hypertensive reactions to tyramine ingested in food	8 - Selective serotonin reuptake inhibitors- Tricyclics- Sympathomimetics
9 - Increased stores of monoamine- Significant accumulation of amine neurotransmitters in the synapses	10 2-3 weeks

1. Which antidepressants may have latency period as short as 48 hours?

2. Which features do MAO inhibitors and tricyclic antidepressants have in common?

3. Tricyclic antidepressants are

4. Which autonomic nervous system effects is common for tricyclic antidepressants?

5. Indicate an effective antidepressant with minimal autonomic toxicity

6. Fluoxetine has fewer adverse effects because of

7. Which tricyclic and heterocyclic antidepressants has the greatest sedation?

8. Which tricyclic and heterocyclic agents has the least sedation?

9. Indicate a tricyclic or a heterocyclic antidepressant having greatest antimuscarinic effects

10. Indicate a tricyclic or a heterocyclic antidepressant having least antimuscarinic effects

1 Tranylcypromine	2 Increase levels of biogenic amines
3 Mixed norepinephrine and serotonin reuptake inhibitors	4 - Antimuscarinic action- Antihistaminic action- Alfa adrenoreceptor-blocking action
5 Fluoxetine	6 Minimal binding to cholinergic, histaminic, and alfa-adrenergic receptors
7 - Doxepin- Amitriptyline- Trazodone	8 Protriptyline
9 Amitriptyline	10 - Trazodone- Buprorion- Mirtazapine

1. Which antidepressants has significant alfa2-adrenoreceptor antagonism?

2. Indicate the main claim for an ideal antidepressant agent

3. Which drugs is least likely to be prescribed to patients with prostatic hypertrophy, glaucoma, coronary and cerebrovascular disease?

4. Indicate the antidepressant agent, which is a phenyltolylpropylamine derivative

5. The mechanism of fluoxetine action includes

6. Which antidepressants is used for treatment of eating disorders, especially buliemia?

7. True or False. Sertaline and paroxetine are similar to fluoxetine in the mechanism of action and therapeutic use, sertaline is less likely to interact adversely with other drugs.

8. A highly selective serotonine reuptake inhibitor is

9. Anxiolytics are used to treat

10. Anxiolytic agents should

1	2
Mirtazapine	- A faster onset of action- Fewer adverse sedative and autonomic effects- Fewer toxicity when overdoses are taken
3	4
Amitriptyline	Fluoxetine
5	6
- Selective inhibition of serotonine uptake in the CNS- Little effect on central norepinephrine or dopamine function- Minimal binding to cholinergic, histaminic, and alfa-adrenergic receptors	Fluoxetine
7	8
TRUE	- Sertaline- Paroxetine- Fluoxetine
9	10
Neurosis	Reduce anxiety and exert a calming effect

1. Anxiolytics are also useful for

2. Indicate the agents of choice in the treatment of most anxiety states

3. The choice of benzodiazepines for anxiety is based on

4. Which anxiolitics is a benzodiazepine derivative

5. Indicate the benzodiazepine, which has the shortest elimination half-life

6. Which benzodiazepines has the shortest duration of action?

7. Which benzodiazepines is less likely to cause cumulative and residual effects with multiple doses?

8. Anxiolytic dosage reduction is recommended

9. Which benzodiazepines is preferred for elderly patients?

10. Which anxiolytics is preferred in patient with limited hepatic function?

1	2
- Treatment of epilepsy and seizures- Insomnia- Muscle relaxation in specific neuromuscular disorders	Benzodiazepines
3	4
- A relatively high therapeutic index- Availability of flumazenil for treatment of overdose- A low risk of physiologic dependence	Clordiazepoxide
5	6
Triazolam	Triazolam
7	8
Lorazepam	- In patients taking cimetidine- In patients with hepatic dysfunction- In elderly patients
9	10
Triazolam	Buspirone

1. Indicate the mechanism of hypnotic benzodiazepine action	**2.** Which anxiolytics is a partial agonist of brain 5-HT1A receptors?
3. Indicate the competitive antagonist of BZ receptors	**4.** Indicate the agent, which interferes with GABA binding
5. Antianxiety agents have	**6.** Which disadvantages does not limit using benzodiazepines as antianxiety agents?
7. Indicate the anxiolitic agent, which relieves anxiety without causing marked sedative effects	**8.** Which anxiolytics has minimal abuse liability?
9. In contrast to benzodiazepines, buspirone	**10.** Which sedative-hypnotic drugs does not potentiate the CNS depressant effects of ethanol, phenothiazines, or tricyclic antidepressants?

1 Increasing the frequency of Cl- channel opening events	2 Buspirone
3 Flumazenil	4 Bicuculline
5 - Sedative and hypnotic activity- Muscle relaxing and anticonvulsant effects- Amnesic properties	6 A high risk of drug interactions based on liver enzyme induction
7 Buspirone	8 Buspirone
9 Causes less psychomotor impairment and does not affect driving skills	10 Buspirone

1 Limitation of buspirone is	2 Which drugs may be used as antianxiety agents?
3 Which benzodiazepines is more likely to cause "hangover" effects such as drowsiness, dysphoria, and mental or motor depression the following day?	4 Additive CNS depression can be predicted if benzodiazepines are used with
5 Which dosage of benzodiazepines for 60-90 days may produce severe withdrawal symptoms?	6 Restlessness, anxiety, orthostatic hypotension, generalized seizures, severe tremor, vivid hallucination, and psychosis are possible symptoms of
7 Flumazenil given intravenously	8 Agents, stimulating CNS are
9 Which CNS stimulants are the agents of selective effect?	10 Indicate CNC stimulating drugs, which are the agents of general action

1 An extremely slow onset of action	2 - BETA-blocking drugs- Clonidine - a partial agonist of alfa2 receptors- Tricyclic antidepressants
3 Clorazepat	4 - Ethanol- Morphine- Clorpromazine
5 50-60 mg/d	6 Withdrawal
7 Acts rapidly but has a short half-life	8 - Fluoxetine- Nootropil- Sydnocarb
9 Psychostimulants	10 Analeptics

1 Which agents belongs to psychostimulants?	**2** Indicate the nootropic agent
3 Which agents is a respiratory analeptic?	**4** Indicate the CNC stimulating drug, which belongs to adaptogens
5 Actoprotectors are	**6** Adaptogens cause
7 Indicate the CNS stimulants, which mitigate conditions of weakness or lack of tone within the entire organism or in particular organs?	**8** Which agents is a general tone-increasing drug of plant origin?
9 Indicate a general tone-increasing drug, which is an agent of animal origin?	**10** Amphetamine

1 Meridil	2 Piracetam
3 Bemegride	4 Eleuterococci extract
5 Stimulators, improving physical efficiency	6 Increased resistance towards stress situations and adaptation to extreme conditions
7 General tonics	8 Eleuterococci's extract
9 Pantocrin	10 - Is a powerful stimulant of the CNS. Stimulates the medullar respiratory center and has an analeptic action. Increases motor and speech activity, mood, decreases a sense of fatigue

1. The mechanism of amphetamine action is related to

2. Indicate the CNS stimulant, which is a piperidine derivative

3. Which CNS psychostimulants is a sydnonymine derivative?

4. Sydnocarb causes

5. Indicate the psychostimulant, which is a methylxantine derivative

6. Which of the following psychostimulants acts centrally mainly by blocking adenosine receptors?

7. Principal properties of caffeine do not include

8. Caffeine can produce

9. Caffeine can not produce

10. Caffeine does not cause

1 - Direct catecholamiergic agonist action - Inhibition of monoamine oxydase - Increasing a release of catecholaminergic neurotransmitters	**2** Meridil
3 Sydnocarb	**4** Decreased sense of fatigue, it facilitates the professional work and fights somnolence
5 Caffeine	**6** Caffeine
7 Adaptogenic (rise non-specific resistance towards stresses and adapt to extraordinary challenges)	**8** - Coronary vasodialation - Relaxation of bronchial and biliary tract smooth muscles - Reinforcement of the contractions and increase of the striaated muscle work
9 Vasodialation of cerebral vessels	**10** Inhibition of gastric secretion

1 Caffeine cause	2 Therapeutic uses of caffeine include
3 Therapeutic uses of caffeine do not include	4 Adverse effects of caffeine include
5 Adverse effects of caffeine do not include	6 Principal properties of cordiamine include
7 Principal properties of cordiamine do not include	8 Characteristics of cordiamine do not include
9 Cordiamine is useful in the treatment of	10 Respiratory and cardiac analeptics are the agents

1 - Hyperglycemia- Moderate diuretic action- Increase in free fatty acids	2 - Cardiovascular collapse and respiratory insufficiency- Migraine- Somnolence
3 Gastric ulceration	4 - Arrhythmias- Insomnia- Psychomotor excitation
5 Hypotension	6 - Cardiac analeptic- Respiratory analeptic- Coronarodilatator
7 Significant abuse potential	8 It decreases the aortic and coronary flow
9 - Hypotension- Coronary insufficiency- Respiratory insufficiency	10 - Cordiamine- Caffeine- Camphor

1	2
Respiratory and cardiac analeptics are not the agents	Bemegride

3	4
Which CNS stimulants belongs to nootropics?	Characteristics of nootropics include

5	6
Characteristics of nootropics do not include	True or False about Nootropics. They improve the highest integrative brain functions (memory, learning, understanding, thinking and the capacity for concentration)

7	8
True or False about Nootropics. They stimulate the bulbar respiratory center	True or False about Nootropics. They stimulate existing neuronal synapses to optimum performance (adaptive capacity)

9	10
Features of piracetam include	Features of piracetam do not include

1	2
Bemegride	Stimulates the medullar respiratory center (central effect)

3	4
Piracetam	- Selective influence on the brain- Improvement the ability to communicate with peers- Increase in energetic exchange of the brain cells

5	6
Decline in the highest integrative brain functions	TRUE

7	8
FALSE	TRUE

9	10
- It is a GABA derivative- It does not influence the neuro-vegetative function- Improvement begins in the 3'rd week	It has a high potential of toxicity

1. Piracetam can produce

2. Piracetam can not produce

3. Piracetam is widely used for the treatment of

4. Which CNS stimulants is used for the cerebral stroke treatment?

5. Psychologic dependence is

6. Tolerance is associated with

7. Addiction is associated with the existence of

8. Substances causing narco- and glue sniffings are

9. Substances causing narco- and glue sniffings are not

10. Which abused drugs do not belong to sedative agents?

1	2
- Anticonvulsant- Psychometabolic- Antihypoxic	Antipsychotic

3	4
- Senile dementia- Asthenia- Chronic alcoholism	Piracetam

5	6
Compulsive drug-seeking behavior	- An ability to compensate for the drug effect- Increased disposition of the drug after chronic use- Compensatory changes in receptors, effector enzymes, or membrane actions of the drug

7	8
- Psychological dependence- Physiological dependence- Tolerance	- Stimulants- Psychedelics- Sedative drugs

9	10
Antipsychotic drugs	Cannabinoids

1	2
Psychedelics are	Psychedelics are not

3	4
In contrast to morphine, heroin is	True or False. Symptoms of opioid withdrawal begin 8-10 hours after the last dose.

5	6
The acute course of opioid withdrawal may last	Indicate the sedative-hypnotic agent, which has the highest abuse potential

7	8
Characteristics of barbiturate intoxication (2-3 dose) do not include	Barbiturate abstinent syndrome is shown by

9	10
Which tranquilizers belongs to strong euphorizing agents?	Tranquilizers intoxication (5-10 tablets) features include:

1 - LSD- Marijuana- Volatile substances (glues, solvents, volatile nitrites and nitrous oxide)	**2** Cocaine
3 More addictive and fast-acting	**4** TRUE
5 7-10 days	**6** Phenobarbital
7 Perceptual distortion of surroundings, disorders of thinking, behavior	**8** - Crisis by 3 day of abstention- Anxiety, mydriasis, myasthenia, muscular convulsions, vomiting, diarrhea- Psychosis as delirium (color visual and auditory hallucinations)
9 Diazepam	**10** Euphoria, burst of energy, increase in motor activity, wave warmth all over the body

1. Which abused drugs is related to stimulants?

2. Cocaine exerts its central action by

3. "Crack" is a derivative of

4. Which stimulants is related to psychedelics?

5. Cocaine may cause

6. Characteristics of cocaine abstinent syndrome do not include

7. Overdoses of cocaine are usually rapidly fatal from

8. Which agents is related to hallucinogens?

9. LSD produces

10. LSD decreases in brain

1	2
- Cocaine - Amphetamine - Caffeine	Inhibiting dopamine and norepinephrine reuptake
3	4
Cocaine	"ecstasy" (methylenedioxymethamphetamine)
5	6
- Powerful vasoconstrictive reactions resulting in myocardial infarctions - The multiple brain perfusion defects - Spontaneous abortion during pregnancy	Psychosis as color visual and auditory hallucinations (for 3 day)
7	8
- Respiratory depression - Arrhythmias - Seizures	LSD
9	10
- Mood swings - Impaired memory, difficulty in thinking, poor judgment - Perceptual distortion	5-HT2 receptor densities

1. Which agents is related to cannabis?

2. The early stage of cannabis intoxication is characterized by

3. Which physiologic signs is a characteristic of cannabis intoxication?

4. Industrial solvent inhalation causes

5. Indicate the drugs of choice for reversing the withdrawal syndrome

6. The state of "general anesthesia" usually includes

7. Inhaled anesthetics and intravenous agents having general anesthetic properties

8. Indicate the anesthetic, which is an inhibitor of NMDA glutamate receptors:

9. An ideal anesthetic drug would

10. Which general anesthetics belongs to inhalants?

1	2
Hashish	- Euphoria, uncontrolled laugher- Alteration of time sense, depersonalization- Sharpened vision

3	4
Reddening of the conjunctiva	- Quick intoxication, lasting only 5-15 minutes- Euphoria, relaxed "drunk" feeling- Disorientation, slow passage of time and possible hallucinations

5	6
- Benzodiazepines- Neuroleptics- Antidepressants	- Analgesia- Loss of consciousness, inhibition of sensory and autonomic reflexes- Amnesia

7	8
Directly activate GABAA receptors	Ketamine

9	10
- Induces anesthesia smoothly and rapidly and secure rapid recovery- Posses a wide margin of safety- Be devoid of adverse effects	Desfluran

1. Indicate the anesthetic, which is used intravenously

2. Which inhalants is a gas anesthetic?

3. Sevoflurane has largely replaced halothane and isoflurane as an inhalation anesthetic of choice because

4. The limitation of sevoflurane is

5. Which inhalants lacks sufficient potency to produce surgical anesthesia by itself and therefore is commonly used with another inhaled or intravenous anesthetic?

6. Which inhaled anesthetics has rapid onset and recovery?

7. Indicate the inhaled anesthetic, which reduces arterial pressure and heart rate

8. Which inhaled anesthetics causes centrally mediated sympathetic activation leading to a rise in blood pressure and heart rate?

9. Indicated the inhaled anesthetic, which decreases the ventilatory response to hypoxia

10. Which inhaled anesthetics is an induction agent of choice in patient with airway problems?

1	2
Propofol	Nitrous oxide

3	4
- Induction of anesthesia is achieved more rapidly and smoothly- Recovery is more rapid- It has low post- anesthetic organ toxicity	Chemically unstable

5	6
Nitrous oxide	- Nitrous oxide- Desflurane- Sevoflurane

7	8
Halothane	Desflurane

9	10
Nitrous oxide	Halothane

1. Indicate the inhaled anesthetic, which causes the airway irritation

2. Which inhaled anesthetics increases cerebral blood flow least of all?

3. Indicate the inhaled anesthetic, which should be avoided in patients with a history of seizure disorders

4. Which inhaled anesthetics can produce hepatic necrosis?

5. Indicated the inhaled anesthetic, which may cause nephrotoxicity

6. Which inhaled anesthetics decreases metheonine synthase activity and causes megaloblastic anemia?

7. Unlike inhaled anesthetics, intravenous agents such as thiopental, etomidate, and propofol

8. Indicate the intravenous anesthetic, which is an ultra-short-acting barbiturate

9. Indicate the intravenous anesthetic, which is a benzodiazepine derivative

10. Which agents is used to accelerate recovery from the sedative actions of intravenous benzodiazepines?

1 Desflurane	2 Nitrous oxide
3 Enflurane	4 Halothane
5 Soveflurane	6 Nitrous oxide
7 - Have a faster onset and rate of recovery- Provide a state of conscious sedation- Are commonly used for induction of anesthesia	8 Thiopental
9 Midazolam	10 Flumazenil

1. Neuroleptanalgesia has the following properties

2. Neuroleptanalgesia has not the following properties

3. Which intravenous anesthetics has antiemetic actions?

4. Indicate the intravenous anesthetic, which causes minimal cardiovascular and respiratory depressant effects

5. Indicate the intravenous anesthetic, which produces dissociative anesthesia

6. Following drugs directly activate the respiratory center

7. Following drugs do not directly activate the respiratory center

8. The mechanism of Cytiton action is

9. Indicate the drug belonging to antitussives of narcotic type of action

10. Tick out the drug belonging to non-narcotic antitussives

1. - Droperidol and fentanyl are commonly used- It can be used with nitrous oxide to provide neuroleptanesthesia- Confusion and mental depression can occur as adverse effects	2. Hypertension is a common consequence
3. Propofol	4. Etomidate
5. Ketamine	6. - Bemegride- Caffeine- Aethymizole
7. Cytiton	8. The reflex mechanism
9. Aethylmorphine hydrochloride	10. Tusuprex

1. Indicate the expectorant with the reflex mechanism

2. Tick the antitussive agent with a peripheral effect

3. True or False. Chymotrypsin is an agent containing free sulfhydryl groups

4. All of these drugs contain free sulfhydryl groups

5. The following drug do not contain free sulfhydryl groups

6. Which drugs is proteolytic enzyme?

7. That drugs destroy disulfide bonds of proteoglycans, which causes depolymerization and reduction of viscosity of sputum

8. That drugs do not destroy disulfide bonds of proteoglycans, which causes depolymerization and reduction of viscosity of sputum

9. Which of these groups of drugs is used for asthma treatment?

10. Tick the drug belonging to non-selective beta2-adrenomimics

1	2
Derivatives of Ipecacucnha and Thermopsis	Libexine
3	4
TRUE	- Acetylcysteine- Ambroxol- Bromhexin
5	6
Trypsin	Desoxiribonuclease
7	8
- Acetylcysteine- Ambroxol- Bromhexin	Desoxiribonuclease
9	10
- Methylxanthines- M-cholinoblocking agents- Beta2 - stimulants	Isoprenaline

1 Select the side-effect characteristic for non-selective beta2-adrenomimics	**2** Bronchodilator drug related to xanthine
3 Bronchodilator drug belonging to sympathomimics	**4** True or False. The property of prolonged theophyllines is the prevention of night asthmatic attacks.
5 The mechanism of methylxanthines action is	**6** Which M-cholinoblocking agents is used especially as an anti-asthmatic?
7 Indicate the side effect of Theophylline	**8** The following drugs are inhaled glucocorticoids
9 The following drugs are not inhaled glucocorticoids	**10** Drug belonging to membranestabilizing agents

1 Tachycardia	2 Theophylline
3 Ephedrine	4 TRUE
5 Inhibition of the enzyme phosphodiesterase	6 Ipratropium
7 Increased myocardial demands for oxygen	8 - Triamcinolone- Beclometazone- Budesonide
9 Sodium cromoglycate	10 Sodium cromoglycate

1. Drug which is a 5-lipoxygenase inhibitor

2. True or False. Zileutin prevents the production of leukotrienes.

3. Indicate the drug which is a leucotriene receptor antagonist

4. True or False. Zafirlucast prevents aspirin-sensitive asthma.

5. Tick the main approach of peptic ulcer treatment

6. Gastric acid secretion is under the control of

7. Gastric acid secretion is not under the control of

8. Indicate the drug belonging to proton pump inhibitors

9. The following agents intensify the secretion of gastric glands

10. The following agent do not intensify the secretion of gastric glands

1 Zileutin	2 TRUE
3 Zafirlucast	4 TRUE
5 - Neutralization of gastric acid- Eradication of Helicobacter pylori- Inhibition of gastric acid secretion	6 - Histamine- Acetylcholine- Gastrin
7 Serotonin	8 Omeprazole
9 - Gastrin- Histamine- Carbonate mineral waters	10 Pepsin

1. Which drugs is an agent of substitution therapy?

2. Choose the drug which is a H2-receptor antagonist

3. The following drugs are proton pump inhibitors

4. Indicate the drug belonging to M1-cholinoblockers

5. Which drugs may cause reversible gynecomastia?

6. True or False. Cimetidine has no effect on hepatic drug metabolism.

7. Tick the drug forming a physical barrier to HCL and Pepsin

8. Which drug is an analog of prostaglandin E1?

9. Select the drug stimulating the protective function of the mucous barrier and the stability of the mucous membrane against damaging factors

10. True or False. Antacids are weak bases that react with gastric hydrochloric acid to form salt and water.

1 Hydrochloric acid	2 Ranitidine
3 - Pantoprozole- Omeprazole- Rabeprazole	4 Pirenzepin
5 Cimetidine	6 FALSE
7 Sucralfate	8 Misoprostole
9 Misoprostol	10 TRUE

1	2
Antacids drugs	Are not Antacids drugs
3	4
Indicate the drug that cause metabolic alkalosis	Drug that causes constipation
5	6
The following drugs stimulate appetite	The following drugs do not stimulate appetite
7	8
True or False. Ethyl alcohol is an agent decreasing appetite.	Fenfluramine
9	10
The following drugs intensify gastrointestinal motility	The following drugs do not intensify gastrointestinal motility

1	2
- Maalox- Mylanta- Almagel	Misoprostol

3	4
Sodium bicarbonate	Aluminium hydroxide

5	6
- Vitamins- Bitters- Insulin	Fepranone

7	8
FALSE	An anorexigenic agent affecting serotoninergic system

9	10
- Metoclopramide- Domperidone- Cisapride	Papaverine

1. True or False. Metoclopramide is a potent dopamine antagonist.

2. Emetic drug of central action

3. The mechanism of Metoclopramide antiemetic action

4. The emetic agent having a reflex action

5. The following drugs are antiemetics

6. The following drugs are not antiemetics

7. Indicate an antiemetic agent which is related to neuroleptics

8. Drugs that reduces intestinal peristalsis

9. Drugs that does not reduces intestinal peristalsis

10. Indicate the laxative drug belonging to osmotic laxatives

1	2
TRUE	Apomorphine hydrochloride

3	4
D2-dopamine and 5-HT3-serotonin receptor blocking effect	Ipecacuanha derivatives

5	6
- Metoclopramide- Ondansetron- Chlorpromazine	Apomorphine hydrochloride

7	8
Prochlorperazine	- Loperamide- Methyl cellulose- Magnesium aluminium silicate

9	10
Cisapride	Sodium phosphate

1. The mechanism of stimulant purgatives is

2. Drug irritating the gut and causing increased peristalsis

3. The following drugs stimulate bile production and bile secretion

4. The following drugs do not stimulate bile production and bile secretion

5. Stimulant of bile production of vegetable origin

6. Select the drug which inhibits peristalsis

7. The drug affecting the biliary system and relaxing Oddy sphincter

8. Drugs thats stimulate erythrogenesis

9. Drugs that does not stimulate erythrogenesis

10. Drug that depressing erythrogenesis

1	2
Increasing motility and secretion	Phenolphthalein
3	4
- Cholenszyme- Oxaphenamide- Cholosas	Chenodiol
5	6
Cholosas	Loperamide
7	8
No-spa	- Iron dextran- Vitamine B12- Folic acid
9	10
Methotrexate	Radioactive phosphorus 32

1. Which drug does not influence leucopoiesis?

2. True or False. Iron deficiency anemia leads to pallor, fatigue, dizziness, exertional dyspnea and other symptoms of tissue ischemia.

3. Drugs used for iron deficiency anemia

4. Drugs that are not used for iron deficiency anemia

5. The drug for parenteral iron therapy

6. Indicate the drug which increases absorption of iron from intestine

7. Pernicious anemia is developed due to deficiency of

8. Drug used for pernicious anemia

9. An adverse effect of oral iron therapy is

10. Drug which contains cobalt atom

1	2
Erythropoetin	TRUE

3	4
- Ferrous sulfate- Ferrous gluconate- Ferrous fumarate	Folic acid

5	6
Fercoven	Ascorbic acid

7	8
Vitamin B12	Cyanocobalamin

9	10
Constipation	Cyanocobalamine

1. Drug used in aplastic anemia	2. True or False. Folic acid is recommended for treatment of megaloblastic anemia.
3. Drug of granulocyte colony-stimulating factor	4. Physiologic reactions are involved in the control of bleeding
5. Physiologic reactions that are not involved in the control of bleeding	6. Which substances is synthesized within vessel walls and inhibits thrombogenesis?
7. The following groups of drugs are for thrombosis treatment	8. The following group of drugs are not for thrombosis treatment
9. Drug belonging to anticoagulants of direct action	10. Which drugs has low-molecular weight?

1 Epoetin alpha	2 TRUE
3 Filgrastim	4 - Platelet adhesion reaction- Platele release reaction- Triggering of the coagulation process
5 Activation of the antifibrinolytic system	6 Prostacyclin (PGI2)
7 - Anticoagulant drugs- Fibrinolitic drugs- Antiplatelet drugs	8 Antifibrinolitic drugs
9 Heparin	10 Enoxaparin

1. Indicate the drug belonging to antagonists of heparin

2. Drug used as an oral anticoagulant

3. Drugs are indirect acting anticoagulants

4. Drugs that are not indirect acting anticoagulants

5. Which drugs belongs to coumarin derivatives?

6. True or False. Heparin is effective when administred orally.

7. Drugs that are antiplatelet agents

8. Drugs that are not antiplatelet agents

9. True or False. The use of heparin is recommended for treatment of deep venous thrombosis.

10. Mechanism of aspirin action is

1 Protamine sulfate	2 Dicumarol
3 - Dicumarol - Warfarin - Phenindione	4 Dalteparin
5 Warfarin	6 FALSE
7 - Aspirin - Ticlopidine - Clopidogrel	8 Urokinase
9 TRUE	10 Inhibits COX and thus thromboxane synthesis

1. Which doses of Aspirin may be more effective in inhibiting Tromboxane A2? (Low or High)

2. Which drugs is an inhibitor of platelet glycoprotein IIb/IIIa receptors?

3. True or False. Ticlopidine is an inhibitor of ADP-induced platelet aggregation.

4. Which drugs is fiibrinolytic?

5. True or False. Mechanism of urokinase action is an inhibition of Thromboxane A2.

6. Fibrinolytic drugs are used for

7. Fibrinolytic drugs are NOT used for

8. Indicate the drug belonging to fibrinoliytic inhibitors

9. Aminocapronic acid is a drug of choice for treatment of

10. True or False. Tranexamic acid is an analog of aminocapronic acid.

1	2
LOW	Abciximab

3	4
TRUE	Streptokinase

5	6
FALSE	- Central deep venous thrombosis- Multiple pulmonary emboli- Acute myocardial infarction

7	8
Heart failure	Aminocapronic acid

9	10
Bleeding from fibrinolytic therapy	TRUE

1	2
Normally involved in the pathogenesis of heart failure	Not Normally involved in the pathogenesis of heart failure
3	4
All of the following are compensatory mechanisms that occur during the pathogenesis of congestive heart failure	The following are not compensatory mechanisms that occur during the pathogenesis of congestive heart failure
5	6
All of the following are recommended at the initial stages of treating patients with heart failure	The following are not recommended at the initial stages of treating patients with heart failure
7	8
The following agents belong to cardiac glycosides	The following agent do not belong to cardiac glycosides
9	10
The non-glycoside positive inotropic drug is	Sugar molecules in the structure of glycosides influence

1 - A cardiac lesion that impairs cardiac output - An increase in peripheral vascular resistance - An increase in sodium and water retention	2 A decrease in preload
3 - An increase in ventricular end-diastolic volume - An increase in the concentration of plasma catecholamines - Increased activity of the renin-angiotensin-aldosterone system	4 An increase in vagal tone
5 - Reduced salt intake - ACE inhibitors - Diuretics	6 Verapamil
7 - Digoxin - Strophantin K - Digitoxin	8 Amrinone
9 Dobutamine	10 Pharmacokinetic properties

1 Aglycone is essential for	**2** Derivative of the plant Foxglove (Digitalis)
3 True or False. They inhibit the Na+/K+-ATPase and thereby increase intracellular Ca++ in myocardial cells	**4** True or False. They cause a decrease in vagal tone
5 True or False. Children tolerate higher doses of digitalis than do adults	**6** True or False. The most frequent cause of digitalis intoxication is concurrent administration of diuretics that deplete K+
7 True or False. An important action of digitalis is to increase vagal tone.	**8** True or False. Digoxin is thought to increase intracellular concentrations of calcium in myocardial cells by indirectly slowing the action of the sodium-calcium exchanger.
9 Compare the half-life of digoxin and the half-life of digitoxin	**10** True or False about cardiac glycosides. They inhibit the activity of the Na+/K+-ATPase

1 Cardiotonic action	2 Digoxin
3 TRUE	4 FALSE
5 TRUE	6 TRUE
7 TRUE	8 TRUE
9 Digitoxin is greater than digoxin	10 TRUE

1. True or False about cardiac glycosides. They decrease intracellular concentrations of calcium in myocytes

2. True or False about cardiac glycosides. They increase vagal tone

3. True or False about cardiac glycosides. They have a very low therapeutic index

4. True or False about cardiac glycosides. Digoxin is a mild inotrope

5. True or False about cardiac glycosides. Digoxin increases vagal tone

6. True or False about cardiac glycosides. Digoxin has a longer half-life than digitoxin

7. True or False about cardiac glycosides. Digoxin acts by inhibiting the Na+/K+ ATPase

8. The most cardiac manifestation of glycosides intoxication is

9. The manifestations of glycosides intoxication are

10. For digitalis-induced arrhythmias the following drug is favored

1	2
FALSE	TRUE
3	4
TRUE	TRUE
5	6
TRUE	FALSE
7	8
TRUE	- Atrioventricular junctional rhythm- Second-degree atrioventricular blockade- Ventricular tachycardia
9	10
- Visual changes- Ventricular tachyarrhythmias- Gastrointestinal disturbances	Lidocaine

1. In very severe digitalis intoxication the best choice is to use

2. True or False about cardiac glycoside-induced ventricular tachyarrhythmias. Lidocaine is a drug of choice in treatment

3. True or False about cardiac glycoside-induced ventricular tachyarrhythmias. Digibind should be used in life-threatening cases

4. True or False about cardiac glycoside-induced ventricular tachyarrhythmias. They occur more frequently in patients with hyperkalemia than in those with hypokalemia

5. True or False about cardiac glycoside-induced ventricular tachyarrhythmias. They are more likely to occur in patients with a severely damaged heart

6. This drug is a selective beta-1 agonist

7. Tolerance to this inotropic drug develops after a few days

8. This drug inhibits breakdown of cAMP in vascular smooth muscle

9. This drug is useful for treating heart failure because it increases the inotropic state and reduces afterload

10. This drug acts by inhibiting type III cyclic nucleotide phosphodiesterase

1 Digibind (Digoxin immune fab)	2 TRUE
3 TRUE	4 FALSE
5 TRUE	6 Dobutamine
7 Dobutamine	8 Amrinone
9 Amrinone	10 Milrinone

1. True or False about inhibitors of type III phosphodiesterase. They raise cAMP concentrations in cardiac myocytes

2. True or False about inhibitors of type III phosphodiesterase. They reduce afterload

3. True or False about inhibitors of type III phosphodiesterase. They show significant cross-tolerance with beta-receptor agonists

4. True or False about inhibitors of type III phosphodiesterase. They are associated with a significant risk for cardiac arrhythmias

5. The following drugs are used in the treatment of severe congestive heart failure

6. The following drug are not used in the treatment of severe congestive heart failure

7. Drugs most commonly used in chronic heart failure are

8. True or False about angiotensin converting enzyme (ACE) inhibitors. They act by inhibiting the ability of renin to convert angiotensinogen to angiotensin I.

9. True or False about angiotensin converting enzyme (ACE) inhibitors. Enalapril is a prodrug that is converted to an active metabolite

10. True or False about angiotensin converting enzyme (ACE) inhibitors. They reduce secretion of aldosterone

1. TRUE	2. TRUE
3. FALSE	4. TRUE
5. - Digoxin- Dobutamine- Dopamine	6. Verapamil
7. - Cardiac glycosides- Diuretics- Angiotensin-converting enzyme inhibitors	8. FALSE
9. TRUE	10. TRUE

1. True or False about angiotensin converting enzyme (ACE) inhibitors. They can produce hyperkalemia in combination with a potassium-sparing diuretic	2. The following effects of ACE inhibitors may be useful in treating heart failure
3. The following effect of ACE inhibitors may be not useful in treating heart failure	4. True or False about the use of angiotensin-converting enzyme (ACE) inhibitors in the treatment of heart failure. They improve hemodynamics by decreasing afterload
5. True or False about the use of angiotensin-converting enzyme (ACE) inhibitors in the treatment of heart failure. They can increase plasma cholesterol levels	6. This drug is a Class IA antiarrhythmic drug
7. This drug is a Class IC antiarrhythmic drug	8. This drug is a Class II antiarrhythmic drug
9. This drug is a Class III antiarrhythmic drug	10. This drug prolongs repolarization

1	2
TRUE	- They decrease afterload- They reduce reactive myocardial hypertrophy- They increase myocardial beta-1 adrenergic receptor density
3	4
They increase circulating catecholamine levels	TRUE
5	6
FALSE	Quinidine
7	8
- Lidocaine- Flecainide	Propranolol
9	10
Sotalol	Sotalol

1 This drug is a Class IV antiarrhythmic drug	**2** This drug is used in treating supraventricular tachycardias
3 This drug is associated with Torsades de pointes	**4** This drug has beta-adrenergic blocking activity
5 This drug is useful in terminating atrial but not ventricular tachycardias	**6** This is a drug of choice for acute treatment of ventricular tachycardias
7 True or False. The calcium channel blockers have direct negative inotropic effects because they reduce the inward movement of calcium during the action potential.	**8** True or False. Common unwanted effects of the dihydropyridines are due to vasodilation.
9 True or False. Verapamil is a more potent vasodilator than nifedipine.	**10** This drug is contraindicated in patients with moderate to severe heart failure

1 Verapamil	2 Digoxin
3 Sotalol	4 Sotalol
5 Verapamil	6 Lidocaine
7 TRUE	8 TRUE
9 FALSE	10 Verapamil

1

This drug is used intravenously to terminate supraventricular tachycardias

2

This drug has a little or no direct effect on chronotropy and dromotropy at normal doses

3

True or False. Verapamil has a significant effect on automaticity in the SA node.

4

This drug acts by inhibiting slow calcium channels in the SA and AV nodes

5

True or False about verapamil. It blocks L-type calcium channels

6

True or False about verapamil. It increases heart rate

7

True or False about verapamil. It relaxes coronary artery smooth muscle

8

True or False about verapamil. It depresses cardiac contractility

9

The following calcium channel blockers are useful in the treatment of cardiac arrhythmias

10

The following calcium channel blockers are not useful in the treatment of cardiac arrhythmias

1 Verapamil	2 Nifedipine
3 TRUE	4 Diltiazem
5 TRUE	6 FALSE
7 TRUE	8 TRUE
9 - Bepridil- Diltiazem- Verapamil	10 Nifedipine

1. The following are common adverse effects of calcium channel blockers

2. The following are not common adverse effects of calcium channel blockers

3. The adverse reactions characteristic for lidocaine

4. True or False about nitrate mechanism of action. Therapeutically active agents in this group are capable of releasing nitric oxide (NO) in to vascular smooth muscle target tissues.

5. True or False about nitrate mechanism of action. Nitric oxide (NO) is an effective activator of soluble guanylyl cyclase and probably acts mainly through this mechanism

6. Which nitrates and nitrite drugs are long-acting?

7. Which nitrates and nitrite drugs is a short-acting drug?

8. Which nitrates and nitrite drugs is used for prevention of angina attack?

9. Duration of nitroglycerin action (sublingual) is

10. True or False about the mechanism of nitrate beneficial clinical effect. Decreased myocardial oxygen requirement

1	2
- Dizziness - Headache - Flushing	Skeletal muscle weakness

3	4
Hypotension, paresthesias, convulsions	TRUE

5	6
TRUE	Sustac

7	8
Amyl nitrite, inhalant (Aspirols, Vaporole)	- Nitroglycerin, 2% ointment (Nitrol) - Nitroglycerin, oral sustained-release (Nitrong) - Isosorbide mononitrate (Ismo)

9	10
10-30 minutes	TRUE

1. True or False about the mechanism of nitrate beneficial clinical effect. Relief of coronary artery spasm

2. True or False about the mechanism of nitrate beneficial clinical effect. Improved perfusion to ischemic myocardium

3. True or False about the mechanism of nitrate beneficial clinical effect. Increased myocardial oxygen consumption

4. Side effect of nitrates and nitrite drugs are

5. True or False about mechanism of calcium channel blockers' action. Calcium channel blockers bind to L-type calcium channel sites

6. Which antianginal agents is a calcium channel blocker?

7. Which cardiovascular system effects refers to a calcium channel blocker?

8. Main clinical use of calcium channel blockers is

9. Which antianginal agents is a myotropic coronary dilator

10. Which antianginal agents is a beta-adrenoceptor-blocking drug

1 TRUE	2 TRUE
3 FALSE	4 - Orthostatic hypotension, tachycardia- Throbbing headache- Tolerance
5 TRUE	6 Nifedipine
7 - The reduction of peripheral vascular resistance- The reduction of cardiac contractility and, in some cases, cardiac output- Relief of coronary artery spasm	8 - Angina pectoris- Hypertension- Supraventricular tachyarrhythmias
9 Dipyridamole	10 Atenolol

1 The following agents are cardioselective beta1-adrenoceptor-blocking drugs labeled for use in angina	2 The following agents are not cardioselective beta1-adrenoceptor-blocking drugs labeled for use in angina
3 True or False about beta-adrenoceptor-blocking drugs. These agents has a moderate reflex and vascular dilative action caused by the stimulation of sensitive nerve endings	4 Which antianginal agents refers to reflex coronary dilators:
5 True or False about Validol. Validol has a moderate reflex and vascular dilative action caused by the stimulation of sensitive nerve endings	6 True or False about Validol. At sublingual administration the effect is produced in five minutes and 70 % of the preparation is released in 3 minutes
7 True or False about Validol. It is used in cases of angina pectoris, motion sickness, nausea, vomiting when seasick or airsick and headaches due to taking nitrates	8 Which antianginal agents is the specific bradycardic drug
9 True or False about Alinidine. Bradycardic drugs have a moderate reflex and vascular dilative action caused by the stimulation of sensitive nerve endings	10 True or False about Alinidine. The predominant effect of bradycardic drugs is a decrease in heart rate without significant changes in arterial pressure

1. Metoprolol- Talinolol- Atenolol	2. Propranolol
3. TRUE	4. Validol
5. TRUE	6. TRUE
7. TRUE	8. Alinidine
9. FALSE	10. TRUE

1. True or False about Alinidine. The protective effect of bradycardic drugs is likely due to a reduced O2 demand

2. True or False about Alinidine. Specific bradycardic agents are used in the management of a wide range of cardiovascular disorders, including sinus tachyarrhythmias and angina pectoris

3. True or False about Dipyridamole. Dipyridamole is an agent that blocks the reabsorption and breakdown of adenosine that results in an increase of endogenous adenosine and vasodilatation

4. True or False about Dipyridamole. The drug causes relative hypoperfusion of myocardial regions served by coronary arteries with haemodynamically significant stenoses

5. True or False about Dipyridamole. Dipyridamole is a platelet aggregation inhibitor

6. Which antianginal agents is a potassium channel opener

7. True or False about potassium channel openers. These agents has a moderate reflex and vascular dilative action caused by the stimulation of sensitive nerve endings

8. This drug reduces blood pressure by acting on vasomotor centers in the CNS

9. The following are central acting antihypertensive drugs

10. A ganglioblocking drug for hypertension treatment is

1. TRUE

2. TRUE

3. TRUE

4. TRUE

5. TRUE

6. Minoxidil

7. FALSE

8. Clonidine

9. - Methyldopa - Clonidine - Moxonidine

10. Trimethaphan

1 A sympatholythic drug	2 Drug with nonselective beta-adrenoblocking activity
3 The selective blocker of beta-1 adrenoreceptors	4 An alpha and beta adrenoreceptors blocker
5 This drug inhibits the angiotensin-converting enzyme	6 This drug is a directly acting vasodilator
7 Diuretic agent for hypertension treatment	8 This drug blocks alpha-1 adrenergic receptors
9 This drug activates alpha-2 adrenergic receptors	10 This drug is an inhibitor of renin synthesis

1 Guanethidine	2 Propranolol
3 Atenolol	4 Labetalol
5 - Captopril - Enalapril - Ramipril	6 Nifedipine
7 Dichlothiazide	8 Prazosin
9 Clonidine	10 Propranolol

1	2
This drug is a non-peptide angiotensin II receptor antagonist	This drug is a potassium channel activator

3	4
True or False about angiotensin II. It is a peptide hormone	True or False about angiotensin II. It stimulates the secretion of aldosterone

5	6
True or False about angiotensin II. Angiotensin I is almost as potent as angiotensin II	True or False about angiotensin II. It is a potent vasoconstrictor

7	8
This drug is contraindicated in patients with bronchial asthma	This drug is converted to an active metabolite after absorption

9	10
This drug routinely produces some tachycardia	True or False about vasodilators. Hydralazine causes tachycardia

1	2
Losartan	Diazoxide

3	4
TRUE	TRUE

5	6
FALSE	TRUE

7	8
Propranolol	Enalapril

9	10
Nifedipine	TRUE

1. True or False about vasodilators. Nifedipine is a dopamine receptor antagonist

2. True or False about vasodilators. Nitroprusside dilates both arterioles and veins

3. True or False about vasodilators. Minoxidil can cause hypertrichosis

4. True or False about verapamil. It blocks L-type calcium channels

5. True or False about verapamil. It increases heart rate

6. True or False about verapamil. It relaxes coronary artery smooth muscle

7. True or False about verapamil. It depresses cardiac contractility

8. Unwanted effects of clonidine

9. The reason of beta-blockers administration for hypertension treatment is

10. An endogenous vasoconstrictor that can stimulate aldosterone release from suprarenal glands

1. FALSE	2. TRUE
3. TRUE	4. TRUE
5. FALSE	6. TRUE
7. TRUE	8. Sedative and hypnotic effects
9. Decreasing of heart work	10. Angiotensin II

1 The group of antihypertensive drugs which diminishes the metabolism of bradykinin	**2** Hydralazine (a vasodilator) can produce
3 Vasodilator which releases NO	**4** The reason of diuretics administration for hypertension treatment is
5 Diuretic agent – aldosterone antagonist	**6** Diuretic agent having a potent and rapid effect
7 The main principle of shock treatment is	**8** Drug which increases cardiac output
9 The synthetic vasoconstrictor having an adrenomimic effect	**10** Indicate the vasoconstrictor of endogenous origin

1	2
Angiotensin-converting enzyme inhibitors	Tachycardia, lupus erhythromatosis
3	4
Sodium nitroprusside	Diminishing of blood volume and amount of Na+ ions in the vessels endothelium
5	6
Spironolactone	Furosemide
7	8
To improve the peripheral blood flow	Noradrenalin
9	10
Phenylephrine	Angiotensinamide

1. Which type of receptors can be activated by angiotensinamide

2. General unwanted effects of vasoconstrictors is

3. For increasing blood pressure in case of low cardiac output the following agents must be used

4. Positive inotropic drug of glycoside structure

5. Positive inotropic drug of non-glycoside structure

6. Dopamine at low doses influences mainly

7. Dopamine at medium doses influences mainly

8. Dopamine in high doses influences mainly the

9. Group of drugs for treatment of shock with hypovolaemia (reduced circulating blood volume)

10. Group of drugs for chronic hypotension treatment

1	2
Angiotensin's receptors	Decrease of peripheral blood flow
3	4
Positive inotropic drugs	Digoxin
5	6
Dobutamine	Dopamine receptors (leads to vasodilation of renal and mesenterial vessels)
7	8
Beta-1 adrenoreceptors (leads to enhanced cardiac output)	Alfa-adrenoreceptors (leads to peripheral vasoconstriction)
9	10
Plasmoexpanders	Analeptics and tonics

1. Indicate the group of drugs influencing the cerebral flow

2. Grug influencing the blood flow which is related to antiplatelet agents

3. Which drugs is related to anticoagulants and may be useful in disorders of cerebral circulation?

4. Indicate the drugs which are Ca-channel blockers influencing the brain blood flow

5. Indicate the drugs influencing the blood flow in the brain - derivatives of GABA

6. Indicate the drug - Vinca minor alcaloid

7. Drug – a derivative of Ergot

8. Indicate the nootropic agent useful in disorders of brain circulation

9. What is the main action of GABA derivatives in disorders of brain circulation?

10. Appropriate mechanism of vinpocetine action

1 - Ca-channel blockers- Derivatives of GABA- Derivatives of Vinca minor plant	2 Aspirin
3 Heparin	4 Nimodipine, Cinnarizine
5 Aminalon, Picamilon	6 Vinpocetine
7 Nicergoline	8 Pyracetam
9 Stimulation of the metabolic processes in neurons	10 It dilates cerebral vessels and improves blood supply

1 Antiaggregants are used in disorders of brain circulation for	2 Migraine is a disorder connected with
3 True or False. Main agents for acute migraine attack treatment are Ergot and indol derivatives and NSAID's.	4 The following Indol derivative is used for treatment of acute migraine attack
5 The following Ergot derivative is used for treatment of acute migraine attack	6 The derivative of lysergic acid for migraine attack prevention is
7 Hormones are	8 An endocrine drug which is an amino acid derivative
9 An endocrine drug which is a peptide derivative	10 An endocrine drug which is a steroidal derivative

1	2
Improving the microcirculation in cerebral tissue	Dysfunction of regulation of cerebral vessel tonus
3	4
TRUE	Sumatriptan
5	6
Ergotamine	Methysergide
7	8
Products of endocrine gland secretion	Thyroxine
9	10
Oxitocin	Hydrocortisone

1. Hormone analogues are

2. True or False about mechanism of action of hormones. Hormones interact with the specific receptors in the wall of the cells

3. True or False about mechanism of action of hormones. Cyclic AMP acts as a second messenger system

4. True or False about mechanism of action of hormones. They stimulate adenylcyclase enzyme

5. True or False about mechanism of action of hormones. Many hormones owe their effect to primary actions on subcellular membrane.

6. Hypothalamic and pituitary hormones (and their synthetic analogs) have pharmacologic applications in three areas, excet

7. Which hormones is produced by the hypothalamic gland?

8. Which hormones is produced by the anterior lobe of the pituitary?

9. The posterior pituitary does NOT secret

10. The posterior pituitary secret

1 Synthetic compounds, which resemble the naturally occurring hormones	2 FALSE
3 TRUE	4 TRUE
5 TRUE	6 As food supplements
7 Growth hormone-releasing hormone (GHRH)	8 Growth hormone (somatotropin, GH)
9 Growth hormone	10 - Vasopressin- Oxytocin

1. Which organs is a target for prolactin?

2. Which organ hormones is a target for growth hormone (somatotropine, GH)?

3. True or False about growth hormone. It may stimulate the synthesis or release of somatomedins

4. True or False about growth hormone. Low levels of insulin-like growth factor (IGF)-1 are associated with dwarfism

5. True or False about growth hormone. Hypersecretion can result in acromegaly

6. True or False about growth hormone. It is contraindicated in subjects with closed epiphyses

7. adrenocorticotropic hormone (ACTH) include

8. adrenocorticotropic hormone (ACTH) do not include

9. True or False. The hypothalamic control exists for the thyroid gland.

10. Indications of bromocriptine are

1 Mammary gland	**2** Insulin-like growth factors (IGF, somatomedins)
3 TRUE	**4** TRUE
5 FALSE	**6** TRUE
7 - Endogenous ACTH is also called corticotropin- ACTH stimulates the synthesis of corticosteroids- ACTH is most useful clinically as a diagnostic tool in adrenal insufficiency	**8** The oral route is the preferred rout of administration
9 TRUE	**10** - Prolactin-secreting adenomas- Amenorrhea-Galactorrhea-Acromegaly

1 Indications of bromocriptine are not	2 Currently used dopamine agonists decreasing pituitary prolactin secretion are following
3 Indications of oxitocin are	4 Indications of vasopressin are
5 Vasopressin possesses the following	6 Oxytocin produces the following effects
7 Vasopressin causes a pressor effect by	8 True or False. Hypothyroidism is a syndrome resulting from deficiency of thyroid hormones and is manifested largely by a reversible slowing down of all body functions
9 Which hormones is produced by the thyroid gland?	10 Which hormones is produced by the thyroid gland?

1	2
Prolactin deficiency	- Bromocriptine- Cabergoline- Pergolide
3	4
- Labor and augment dysfunctional labor for conditions requiring early vaginal delivery- Incompleted abortion- For control of pospartum uterine hemorrhage	Pituitary diabetes insipidus
5	6
Antidiuretic property	- It causes contraction of the uterus- It assists the progress of spermatozoa into the uterine cavity- It brings about milk ejection from the lactating mammary gland
7	8
A direct action on smooth muscles of the blood vessels	TRUE
9	10
Thyroxine	Triiodothyronine

1. Thyroid stimulating hormone regulates the following

2. True or False about Thyroid hormones. Decline of the basal metabolic rate in the body

3. True or False about Thyroid hormones. Increase in the rate and force of contraction of the heart

4. True or False about Thyroid hormones. Increase in the blood cholestrol level

5. True or False about Thyroid hormones. Increase in the heat production

6. Synthesis and release of thyroid hormones are controlled by

7. Thyrotrophin stimulates

8. The rate of secretion of thyrotropin is controlled by

9. Indications of thyroid hormones are

10. The common side effect of thyroid hormones is

1 - Iodine uptake- Biosynthesis of iodothyroglobulin- Release of thyroid hormone into the plasma	2 FALSE
3 TRUE	4 TRUE
5 TRUE	6 - Anterior pituitary alone- Hypothalamus alone- Blood levels of thyroid hormones alone
7 Release of thyroxine and triidothyronine	8 The concentration of thyroid hormones in blood
9 - Cretinism- Myxoedema- Hashimoto's disease	10 Exopthalmos

1	2
Currently used antithyroid drugs include the following	In an area where goitre is endemic, which of the following drugs is used?

3	4
Iodide preparations can be used in following situations	Iodide preparations can not be used in following situations

5	6
Daily administration of large doses (several milligrammes) of iodides to a thyrotoxic patient causes	Radioiodines (I131 and I132) is suitable for

7	8
Radioiodines in the body emit	Secretory products of pancreatic β-cells are

9	10
Insulin is	Insulin is a polypeptide hence

1 - Propylthiouracil (PTU)- Diatrizoate sodium (Hypaque)- Methimazole (Tapazole)	**2** Iodide 1 part in 100000
3 - In thyroid disorders- In granulomatous lesions e.g. Syphilis- As an antiseptic	**4** In iodism
5 Thyroid gland growing firm and less vascular	**6** Elderly patients (over 45 years)
7 Mainly β radiations	**8** Insulin, C-peptide, proinsulin, islet amyloid polypeptide (IAPP)
9 A small protein with a molecular weight of 5808 having disulphide linkage	**10** It is destroyed by gastric juice

1. True or False. Bovine insulin is less antigenic than porcine.

2. Insulin causes reduction in blood sugar level by the following mechanisms

3. True or False about glucagon. Stimulates gluconeogenesis in the liver

4. Insulin can not be administered by

5. Sources of human insulin production are

6. The primary reason for a physician to prescribe human insulin is that

7. True or False about crystalline zinc (regular) insulin. It can serve as replacement therapy for juvenile-onset diabetes

8. True or False about crystalline zinc (regular) insulin. It can be administered intravenously

9. True or False about crystalline zinc (regular) insulin. It is a short-acting insulin

10. True or False about crystalline zinc (regular) insulin. It can be administered orally

1	2
FALSE	- Increased glucose uptake in the peripheral tissue- Reduction of breakdown of glycogen- Diminished gluconeogenesis
3	4
TRUE	Oral route
5	6
Recombinant DNA techniques by inserting the proinsulin gene into E. coli or yeast	It can be given to patients who have an allergy to animal insulins
7	8
TRUE	TRUE
9	10
TRUE	FALSE

1 Diabetic coma is treated by the administration of	2 Sulphonylureas act by
3 True or False. Sulphonylureas are effective in totally insulin deficient patients.	4 Currently used second-generation sulfonylureas include
5 Currently used oral hypoglycemic thiazolidinediones include	6 Thiazolidinediones act by
7 Currently used alpha-glucosidase inhibitors include	8 Alpha-glucosidase inhibitors act by
9 Potency of action of	10 Which oral hypoglycaemic drugs stimulates both synthesis and release of insulin from beta islet cells

1	2
Crystalline insulin	Stimulating the beta islet cells of pancreas to produce insulin

3	4
FALSE	- Glyburide (Glibenclamide)- Glipizide (Glydiazinamide)- Glimepiride (Amaril)

5	6
- Pioglitazone (Actos)- Rosiglitazone (Avandia)	Diminishing insulin resistance by increasing glucose uptake and metabolism in muscle and adipose tissues

7	8
- Acarbose (Precose)- Miglitol (Glyset)- All of the above	Competitive inhibiting of intestinal alpha-ghucosidases and modulating the postprandial digestion and absorption of starch and disaccharides

9	10
Miglitol is six times higher than that of acarbose	Glibenclamide

1 Currently used oral hypoglycemic biguanides include	2 The action of insulin is potentiated by
3 Duration of action of	4 True or False. Side effects of sulphonylureas are less than those of biguanides.
5 Biguanides are used in	6 Which agents is/are important hormonal antagonists of insulin in the body?
7 Glucagon is	8 True or False. Glucagon is synthesized in the A cells of the pancreatic islets of Langerhans.
9 True or False. Glucagon is a peptide – identical in all mammals – consisting of a single chain of 29 amino acids	10 True or False. Glucagon is extensively degraded in the liver and kidney as well as in plasma, and at its tissue receptor sites.

1 - Repaglinide (Prandin)- Metformin- Phenformine	2 Biguanides
3 Chlorpropamide is more than that of tolbutamide	4 TRUE
5 In case of hyperglycemic shock	6 - Glucagon- Adrenal steroids- Adrenaline
7 A peptide – identical in all mammals – consisting of a single chain of 29 amino acids.	8 TRUE
9 TRUE	10 TRUE

1. True or False. Half-life of glucagon is between 6 and 8 hours, which is similar to that of insulin.

2. Glucagon can be used in

3. Main complications of insulin therapy include

4. The major natural estrogens produced by women are

5. True or False. Estrogens are required for normal sexual maturation and growth of the female

6. True or False. Estrogens decrease the rate of resorption of bone

7. True or False. Estrogens enhance the coagulability of blood

8. The major synthetic estrogens are

9. True or False about estrogens. Estradiol binds strongly to an α2-globulin and albumin with lower affinity

10. True or False about estrogens. Estrone and estriol have lower affinity for the estrogen receptors than estradiol

1 FALSE	2 - Severe hypoglycemia - Endocrine diagnosis - Beta-blocker poisoning
3 - Hypoglycemia - Insulin allergy - Lipodystrophy at an injection site	4 - Estradiol (Estradiol-17β, E2) - Estron (E1) - Estriol (E3)
5 TRUE	6 TRUE
7 TRUE	8 - Dienestrol - Diethylstilbestrol - Benzestrol
9 TRUE	10 TRUE

1. Indications of synthetic estrogens are

2. Main complications of estrogens' therapy include

3. Main contraindications of estrogens' therapy include

4. Tamoxifen is

5. Progesterone is secreted by

6. The major natural progestin is

7. True or False about progestins. Progesterone is rapidly absorbed following administration by any route

8. True or False about progestins. In the liver, progesterone is metabolized to pregnanediol and conjugated with glucuronic acid.

9. True or False about progestins. Significant amounts of progestins and their metabolites are excreted in the urine

10. True or False. The normal ovary produces small amount of androgens, including testosterone, androstenedione, and degydroepiandrosterone.

1	2
- Primary hypogonadism- Postmenopausal hormonal therapy- Hormonal contraception	- Postmenopausal uterine bleeding- Breast tenderness- Hyperpigmentation
3	4
- Estrogen-dependent neoplasmas such as carcinoma of the endometrium or carcinoma of the breast- Undiagnosed genital bleeding- Liver disease	Antiestrogen
5	6
Corpus luteum	Progesterone
7	8
TRUE	TRUE
9	10
TRUE	TRUE

1	2
Noncontraceptive clinical uses of progestins are	True or False. Estrogens possess immunomodulator properties, but progestins do immunodepressant ones.
3	4
Mifepristone (RU-486) is	True or False. Mifepristone (RU-486) is used as a contraceptive and abortifacient.
5	6
True or False about oral contraceptives. The "combination pill" contains both estrogen and progestin	True or False about oral contraceptives. Ethinyl estradiol and mestranol are commonly used in oral contraceptives
7	8
True or False about oral contraceptives. The "minipill" contains progestin alone	True or False about oral contraceptives. The "triphasic pill" contains estrogen, progestin, and luteinizing hormine (LH)
9	10
Glucocorticoids are hormonal steroids	Inflammation is

1 - Hormone replacement therapy- Dysmenorrhea- Endometriosis	2 TRUE
3 Antiprogestin	4 TRUE
5 TRUE	6 TRUE
7 TRUE	8 FALSE
9 Having an important effect on intermediary metabolism, cardiovascular function, growth, and immunity	10 A localized protective reaction of a tissue to irritation, injury, or infection, characterized by pain, redness, swelling, and sometimes loss of function

1	2
An acute, transient phase, of inflammation is characterized by	A delayed, subacute phase, of inflammation is characterized by
3	4
A chronic, proliferative phase, of inflammation is characterized by	The following substances are considered to be referred to as eicosanoids
5	6
True or False about cortisol (hydrocortisone). Cortisol is synthesized from cholesterol	True or False about cortisol (hydrocortisone). ACTH governs cortisol secretion
7	8
True or False about cortisol (hydrocortisone). Most cortisol is inactivated in the liver	True or False about cortisol (hydrocortisone). The half-life of cortisol in the circulations is normally about 60-90 hours.
9	10
True or False about glucocorticoids. Effects of glucocorticoids are mediated by widely distributed glucocorticoid receptors that are members of the superfamily of nuclear receptors.	True or False about glucocorticoids. Glucocorticoids have dose-related metabolic effects on carbohydrate, protein, and fat metabolism.

1	2
Local vasodilatation and increased capillary permeability (phase of damage)	Infiltration of leucocytes and phagocytic cells (phase of exudation)
3	4
Tissue degeneration and fibrosis occurrence (phase of proliferation)	- Prostaglandins- Leukotrienes- Thromboxanes
5	6
TRUE	TRUE
7	8
TRUE	FALSE
9	10
TRUE	TRUE

1. True or False about glucocorticoids. Glucocorticoids have pro-inflammatory effects.

2. True or False about glucocorticoids. Glucocorticoids have catabolic effects in lymphoid and connective tissue, muscle, fat, and skin.

3. Which glucocorticoids is a short- to medium-acting drug?

4. Which glucocorticoids is an intermediate-acting drug?

5. Which glucocorticoids is a long-acting drug?

6. Which glucocorticoids have one fluoride atom in its chemical structure?

7. Which glucocorticoids have two fluoride atoms in its chemical structure?

8. Which glucocorticoids has no fluoride atoms in its chemical structure?

9. Anti-inflammatory effect of glucocorticoids is caused by

10. True or False about anti-inflammatory effect of glucocorticoids. Anti-inflammatory effect of glucocorticoids results from inhibition of cyclooxygenase

1	2
FALSE	TRUE
3	4
Prednisolon	Triamcinolone
5	6
Dexamethasone	Triamcinolone
7	8
Fluocinolone	Prednisolon
9 - Reducing the prostaglandin and leukotriene which results from inhibition of phospholipase A2- Reducing macrophages migration into the site of inflammation- Decreasing capillary permeability	10 FALSE

1. Immunosupressive effect of glucocorticoids is caused by

2. True or False about anti-inflammatory effect of NSAIDs. Anti-inflammatory effect of NSAIDs results from inhibition of cyclooxygenase

3. True or False about anti-inflammatory effect of NSAIDs. Anti-inflammatory effect of NSAIDs results from inhibition of phospholipase A2 and reducing prostaglandin and leukotriene synthesis

4. Serious side effects of glucocorticoids include

5. Serious side effects of glucocorticoids include

6. True or False. Selective COX-2 inhibitors are safer than nonselective COX-1 inhibitors but without loss of efficacy.

7. True or False. The constitutive COX-2 isoform tends to be homeostatic in function, while COX-1 is induced during inflammation and tends to facilitate the inflammatory response.

8. Which property combinations is peculiar to the majority of NSAIDs?

9. Which NSAIDs is a propionic acid derivative?

10. Which NSAIDs is an indol derivative?

1. Reducing concentration of lymphocytes (T and B cells) and inhibiting function of tissue macrophages and other antigen-presenting cells	2. TRUE
3. FALSE	4. - Acute peptic ulcers- Iatrogenic Cushing's syndrome (rounding, puffiness, fat deposition and plethora alter the appearance of the face – moon faces)- Hypomania or acute psychosis
5. - Adrenal suppression- Insomnia, behavioral changes (primarily hypomania)- Rounding, puffiness, fat deposition and plethora alter the appearance of the face – moon faces	6. TRUE
7. FALSE	8. Antipyretic, analgesic, anti-inflammatory
9. Ibuprofen	10. Indomethacin

1. Which NSAIDs is a pyrazolone derivative?

2. Which NSAIDs is a fenamate derivative?

3. Which NSAIDs is an oxicam derivative?

4. Which NSAIDs is a selective COX-2 inhibitor?

5. Which NSAIDs is a nonselective COX inhibitor

6. True or False. Aspirin inhibits phospholipase A2

7. Side effects of aspirin include

8. Serious side effects of metamizole (analgin) include

9. Side effects of indometacin include

10. True or False. Ketoprofen is a propionic acid derivative that inhibits both cyclooxygenase (nonselectively) and lipoxygenase.

1	2
Metamizole (Analgin)	Meclofenamic acid
3	4
Piroxicam	Celecoxib
5	6
Piroxicam	TRUE
7	8
- Gastric upset (intolerance)- Salicylism (vomiting, tinnitus, decreased hearing, and vertigo)- Gastric ulcers and upper gastrointestinal bleeding	Agranulocytosis, aplastic anemia
9	10
- Abdominal pain, diarrhea, gastrointestinal hemorrhage and pancreatitis- Dizziness, confusion and depression- Trombocytopenia	TRUE

1. True or False. Ketorolac is an NSAID that is promoted for systemic use as an anti-inflammatory, not as an analgesic drug.

2. Which drugs is a 5-lipoxygenase (5-LOG) inhibitor?

3. Which drugs is a leucotreine D4 receptor (LTD4) blocker?

4. Which drugs is a thromboxane A2 receptor (TXA2) antagonist?

5. Adaptive (acquired) immunity refers to

6. Allergic reaction is

7. Immediate allergy reaction (type I allergic reaction) is

8. Delayed allergy reaction (type IV allergic reaction) is

9. Immunodeficiency

10. H1 histamine receptor subtype is distributed in

1 FALSE	2 Zileuton (Zyflo)
3 Zafirleukast (Accolate)	4 Sulotroban
5 Antigen-specific defense mechanisms that take several days to become protective and are designed to react with and remove a specific antigen. This is the immunity one develops throughout life	6 A local or generalized reaction of an organism to internal or external contact with a specific allergen to which the organism has been previously sensitized
7 An allergic or immune response that begins within a period lasting from a few minutes to about an hour after exposure to an antigen to which the individual has been sensitized	8 An allergic reaction that becomes apparent only hours after contact
9 A disorder or deficiency of the normal immune response	10 Smooth muscle, endothelium and brain

1 H2 histamine receptor subtype is distributed in	**2** Most tissue histamine is sequestered and bound in
3 These categories of histamine H1 antagonists are noted for sedative effects	**4** Which category of histamine H1 antagonists is noted for the best antiemetic action?
5 These categories of histamine H1 antagonists are noted for the anticholinergic effect	**6** Which category of histamine H1 antagonists is noted for the alpha-adrenoreceptor-blocking effect?
7 Which category of histamine H1 antagonists is noted for the highest local anesthetic effect?	**8** Which category of histamine H1 antagonists is recognized for as second-generation antihistamines?
9 These histamine H1 antagonists are recognized for as second-generation antihistamines	**10** Which of histamine H1 antagonists is noted for the serotonin-blocking effect?

1 Gastric mucosa, cardiac muscle, mast cells and brain	2 - Granules in mast cells or basophils- Cell bodies of histaminergic neurons- Enterochromaffin-like cell of the fondus of the stomach
3 - Ethanolamines (aminoalkyl ethers), i.e. Dimedrol, Clistin- Ethylenediamines, i.e. Suprastine- Phenothiazines, i.e. Diprazine, Promethazine	4 Ethanolamines (aminoalkyl ethers), i.e. Doxylamine
5 - Alkylamines (propylamines), i.e. Brompheniramine- Ethylenediamines, i.e. Suprastine- Phenothiazines, i.e. Diprazine, Promethazine	6 Phenothiazines, i.e. Diprazine, Promethazine
7 Phenothiazines, i.e. Promethazine	8 Piperidines, i.e. Loratadine, Fexofenadine
9 - Astemizole- Loratadine (Claritin)- Cetirizine (Zyrtec)	10 Cyproheptadine

1. Which histamine H1 antagonists is a long-acting (up to 24-48 h) antihistamine drug?

2. Which of histamine H1 antagonists is noted for the ulcerogenic effect?

3. Indication for administration of histamine H1 antagonists is

4. Indications for administration of histamine H1 antagonists are

5. Side effect of first-generation histamine H1 antagonists is

6. Immunosupressive effect of glucocorticoids is caused by

7. The Immunosuppressive agent is

8. Class of cyclosporine A is

9. Mechanism of action of cyclosporine A is

10. Side effect of cyclosporine A is

1 Diazoline	2 Diazoline
3 - Prevention or treatment of the symptoms of allergic reactions (rhinitis, urticaria)- Motion sickness and vestibular disturbances- Nausea and vomiting in pregnancy ("morning sickness")	4 - Prevention or treatment of the symptoms of allergic reactions (rhinitis, urticaria)- Nausea and vomiting in pregnancy ("morning sickness")- Treatment of sleep disorders
5 Sedation	6 Reducing concentration of lymphocytes (T and B cells) and inhibiting function of tissue macrophages andother antigen-presenting cells
7 - Corticosteroids- Cyclosporine- Tacrolimus (FK 506)	8 Immunosuppressive agents
9 Inhibits calcineurin	10 - Tremor- GI disturbance- Hepatotoxicity

1	2
Side effect of cyclosporine A is	Side effect of cyclosporine A is

3	4
Indication of cyclosporine A is	Half-life of cyclosporine A is

5	6
Class of I.V. IgG preparation is	Mechanism of action of I.V. IgG preparation is

7	8
Half-life of I.V. IgG preparation is:	Indication for I.V. IgG preparation administration is

9	10
Cytotoxic agents are	Class of sirolimus (rapamycin) is

1 Tremor	2 GI disturbance
3 Idiopathic nephrotic syndrome	4 19 hours
5 Immunoglobulins	6 Compete for Fc receptors with autoantibodies
7 21 days	8 Prophylaxis of certain infections
9 - Azathioprine- Leflunomide- Cyclophosphamide	10 Immunosuppressive agents

1	2
Mechanism of action of sirolimus (rapamycin) is	Monoclonal antibodies is

3	4
Class of OKT-3 is	Half-life of OKT-3 is

5	6
The indication for interferon gamma administration is	The side effect of interferon gamma is

7	8
Half-life of interferon gamma is	Half-life of interferon alpha is

9	10
The indication for interferon alpha administration is	Class of tacrolimus (FK-506) is

1	2
Inhibits calcineurin	- Trastuzumab - Rituximab - OKT-3

3	4
Monoclonal antibodies	18-24 hours

5	6
Chronic granulomatous disease	Fatigue

7	8
25-35 minutes	4-16 hours

9	10
- Hepatitis C virus infection - Kaposi's sarcoma - Condyloma acuminatum	Immunosuppressive agents

1 Mechanism of action of tacrolimus (FK-506) is	2 Immunomodulating agent is
3 Immunomodulating agents are	4 Mechanism of action of levamisole is
5 Vitamins are	6 Vitamin-like compounds are
7 Antivitamins are	8 Coenzymes are
9 Antienzymes are	10 True or False. Hypovitaminosis is an insufficiency of one or more essential vitamins.

1 Inhibits calcineurin	2 Levamisole
3 Tacrolimus (FK-506)	4 Increase the number of T-cells
5 Any of various fat-soluble or water-soluble organic substances essential in minute amounts for normal growth and activity of the body and obtained naturally from plant and animal fo	6 A number of compounds, whose nutritional requirements exist at specific periods of development, particularly neonatal development, and periods of rapid growth
7 Substances that prevent vitamins from exerting their typical metabolic effects	8 Nonprotein organic substances that usually contain a vitamin or mineral and combines with a specific apoenzyme to form an active enzyme system
9 Agents, especially an inhibitory enzymes or an antibodies to enzymes, that retard, inhibit, or destroy enzymic activity	10 TRUE

1 Select a fat-soluble vitamin	**2** Select a water-soluble vitamin
3 Which vitamins can be also synthesized from a dietary precursor?	**4** Which vitamins resembles with hormone
5 Beri-beri is caused by the deficiency of	**6** True or False about vitamin A functions. Retinoic acid is especially important during embryogenesis
7 True or False about vitamin A functions. Acts as a hormone involved in regulation of calcium and phosphorus homeostasis	**8** Xerophthalmia is
9 Keratomalacia is:	**10** Night blindness (Hemeralopia, Nyctalopia) is

1 Tocopherol	2 Vitamin B1
3 Vitamin A	4 Vitamin D
5 Thiamine	6 TRUE
7 FALSE	8 Extreme dryness of the conjunctiva resulting from a disease localized in the eye or from systemic deficiency of vitamin A
9 A condition, usually in children with vitamin A deficiency, characterized by softening and subsequent ulceration and perforation of the cornea	10 A condition of the eyes in which vision is normal in daylight or other strong light but is abnormally weak or completely lost at night or in dim light and that results from vitamin A deficiency

1. True or False about vitamin E functions. Antisterility and antiabortion factor	2. True or False about vitamin E functions. Specifically required for synthesis of prothrombin and several other clotting factors
3. True or False about vitamin E functions. An essential for oxidative processes regulation	4. True or False about vitamin B1. An essential coenzyme for oxidative decarboxylate of alpha-keto acids, most important being conversion of pyruvate to acetyl coenzyme A
5. True or False about vitamin B2 functions. Essential constituent of flavoproteins, flavin mononucleotide (FMN) and flavin adenine dinucleotide (FAD)	6. True or False about vitamin B2 functions. Plays key roles in hydrogen transfer reactions associated with glycolysis, TCA cycle and oxidative phosphorylation
7. True or False about vitamin B2 functions. An essential coenzyme for oxidative decarboxylate of alpha-keto acids, most important being conversion of pyruvate to acetyl coenzyme A	8. True or False about vitamin B2 functions. Deficiency symptoms are cheilitis, cheilosis and angular stomatitis
9. True or False about vitamin PP (B3, niacin) functions. Active group of the coenzymes nicotinamide-adenine dinucleotide (NAD) and nicotinamide-adenine phosphate (NADP)	10. True or False about pantothinic acid functions. Essential constituent of coenzyme A, the important coenzyme for acyl transfer in the TCA cycle and de novo fatty acid synthesis

1 TRUE	2 FALSE
3 TRUE	4 TRUE
5 TRUE	6 TRUE
7 FALSE	8 TRUE
9 TRUE	10 TRUE

1. True or False about vitamin C functions. Has antioxidant properties and is required for various hydroxylation reactions e.g. proline to hydroxypoline for collagen synthesis	**2.** Dermatitis, diarrhoea and dementia are characteristics of
3. Pellagra is	**4.** Rickets is
5. Scurvy is	**6.** Which vitamins is given along with isoniazide in treatment of tuberculosis?
7. Which vitamins is also known as an antisterility factor?	**8.** Mega doses of which vitamin are some time beneficial viral respiratory infections
9. Which vitamins improves megaloblast anemia but does not protect the neurological manifestations of pernicious anemia?	**10.** True or False. Vitamin K enhances the anticoagulant property of coumarins.

1 TRUE	2 Pellagra
3 A disease caused by a deficiency of niacin in the diet and characterized by skin eruptions, digestive and nervous system disturbances, and eventual mental deterioration	4 A deficiency disease resulting from a lack of vitamin D or calcium and from insufficient exposure to sunlight, characterized by defective bone growth and occurring chiefly in children
5 A disease caused by deficiency of vitamin C and characterized by spongy bleeding gums, bleeding under the skin, and weakness	6 Pyridoxine
7 Vitamin E	8 Vitamin C
9 Vitamin B12	10 FALSE

1. Loosening of teeth, gingivitis and hemorrhage occur in the deficiency of

2. Ingestion of polar bear liver may cause acute poisoning of

3. Which antivitamins prevent a vitamin B6 from exerting its typical metabolic effects?

4. Which antivitamins prevent a vitamin A from exerting its typical metabolic effects?

5. Which antivitamins prevent a vitamin K from exerting its typical metabolic effects?

6. Which coenzymes is of vitamin origin?

7. Which coenzymes is not of vitamin origin?

8. These substances are vitamin-like compounds

9. Which substances is a vitamin-like compound?

10. Which antienzymes is a proteolysis inhibitor?

1	2
Vitamin C	Vitamin A
3	4
- Isoniazide- Ethanol- Carbamazepine	Lipooxidase
5	6
- Cholestiramine- Coumarins- Antibiotics	Piridixal-5-phosphate
7	8
- Coenzyme Q10- Magnesium- Carnitine	- Choline- Vitamin U (methylmethioninesulfonil chloride)- Orotate acid
9	10
Taurine	Contrical

1. Which antienzymes is a beta-lactamase inhibitor?

2. Which antienzymes is a fibrinolysis inhibitor?

3. Which antienzymes is an aldehyde dehydrogenase inhibitor?

4. Which antienzymes is a cholinesterase inhibitor?

5. Which antienzymes is a monoamine oxidase (MAO) inhibitor

6. Which antienzymes is a xantine oxidase inhibitor?

7. Which antienzymes is an aromatase inhibitor used in cancer therapy?

8. Which enzymes improves GIT functions (replacement therapy)

9. Which enzymes has fibrinolytic activity?

10. Which enzymes is used in cancer therapy?

1	2
- Clavulanic acid- Sulbactam- Tazobactam	Aminocaproic acid

3	4
Disulfiram	Physostigmine

5	6
Selegiline	Allopurinol

7	8
Aminoglutethimide	Pepsin

9	10
Urokinase	L-asparaginase

1. True or False about nutritional supplement (dietary supplement). Nutritional supplements are regulated as foods, and not as drugs

2. True or False about nutritional supplement (dietary supplement). Nutritional supplements are not pre-approved on their safety and efficacy, unlike drugs

3. Lipoprotein is

4. Very low density lipoprotein (VLDL) is

5. Low-density lipoprotein (LDL) is

6. Chylomicron is

7. True or False. Hyperlipoproteinemia is a condition marked by an abnormally high level of lipoproteins in the blood.

8. True or False. Hypercholesterolemia (or hypercholesteremia) is an abnormally high concentration of cholesterol in the blood. This

9. True or False. Familial chylomicronemia (type I) is caused by deficiency in lipoprotein lipase activity.

10. True or False. The Coronary Primary Prevention Trial (CPPT) demonstrated that treatment with a lipid-lowering drug could reduce the risk of death due to coronary heart disease.

1	2
TRUE	TRUE

3	4
A conjugated protein having a lipid component, the principal means for transporting lipids in the blood	A lipoprotein containing a very large proportion of lipids to protein and carrying most cholesterol from the liver to the tissues

5	6
A lipoprotein that contains relatively high amounts of cholesterol and is associated with an increased risk of atherosclerosis and coronary artery disease. It is also called beta-lipoprotein	Large lipoprotein particle that is created by the absorptive cells of the small intestine. It transports lipids to adipose tissue where they are broken down by lipoprotein lipase

7	8
TRUE	TRUE

9	10
TRUE	TRUE

1. True or False. Women taking probucol (Lorelco) should wait for 6 months after cessation of therapy before becoming pregnant.

2. True or False. Nicotinic acid (Niacin) plus a bile acid-binding resin has not proven effective in combating hyperlipidemia.

3. True or False. Agents, which lower levels of LDL-cholesterol, tend to promote regression of atherosclerotic plaques.

4. True or False. Clofibrate (Atromid-S) is the drug of choice for treatment of broad-beta hyperlipidemia (type III).

5. True or False. One advantage of gemfibrozil (Lopid) is that, in addition to lowering blood levels of most lipids, it raises the level of HDL cholesterol.

6. True or False. Probucol (Lorelco) appears to increase clearance of LDL cholesterol by a non-receptor mediated mechanism.

7. True or False about cholestyramine (Questran). It would not be a good choice for treating patients with familial hypertriglyceridemia (type IV)

8. True or False about cholestyramine (Questran). It is not well tolerated by patients

9. True or False about cholestyramine (Questran). It works by directly binding cholesterol in the blood

10. True or False about cholestyramine (Questran). It is an effective drug for treatment of types IIa and IIb hyperlipidemia

1	2
TRUE	FALSE

3	4
TRUE	FALSE

5	6
TRUE	TRUE

7	8
TRUE	TRUE

9	10
FALSE	TRUE

1. True or False about drugs which inhibit cholesterol synthesis. They work in part by increasing the rate of LDL clearance from the plasma

2. True or False about drugs which inhibit cholesterol synthesis. They are the most effective single agents for lowering LDL-cholesterol

3. True or False about drugs which inhibit cholesterol synthesis. When used with a bile-acid binding resin, they can lower LDL-cholesterol by 50% or more

4. True or False about drugs which inhibit cholesterol synthesis. No special monitoring is required in patients receiving one of them

5. True or False about nicotinic acid (Niacin). It reduces the rate of synthesis of VLDL

6. True or False about nicotinic acid (Niacin). Sustained-release preparations of this drug are largely free of side effects

7. True or False about nicotinic acid (Niacin). Almost all patients taking the traditional dosage form of this drug experience uncomfortable flushing

8. True or False about nicotinic acid (Niacin). It should not be used with antihypertensives

9. True or False about drugs which inhibit cholesterol synthesis. When used alone, they are the most effective agents for lowering LDL cholesterol

10. True or False about drugs which inhibit cholesterol synthesis. They are often effective in patients in whom a diet, with or without a bile acid-binding resin or niacin, has failed

1 TRUE	2 TRUE
3 TRUE	4 FALSE
5 TRUE	6 FALSE
7 TRUE	8 TRUE
9 TRUE	10 TRUE

1. True or False about drugs which inhibit cholesterol synthesis. Lovastatin (Mevacor) plus a resin causes regression of coronary lesions in about one third of treated patients

2. True or False about drugs which inhibit cholesterol synthesis. Members of this drug class are generally not as well tolerated as the older bile acid-binding resins

3. True or False about drugs which inhibit cholesterol synthesis. These drugs should not be used in pregnant women or children

4. True or False about drugs which inhibit cholesterol synthesis. These drugs often cause myopathy if used in combination with cyclosporine (Sandimmune)

5. True or False about drugs which inhibit cholesterol synthesis. Failure to discontinue the drug after myopathy has been detected can cause acute renal failure

6. True or False about drugs which inhibit cholesterol synthesis. Several of these drugs tend to lengthen the sleep cycle

7. True or False about the fibric acid derivatives. Clofibrate (Atromid-S) is the drug of choice for therapy of Type III hyperlipidemia

8. True or False about the fibric acid derivatives. Gemfibrozil (Lopid) increases HDL cholesterol while lowering LDL cholesterol

9. True or False about the fibric acid derivatives. Gemfibrozil (Lopid) has been shown to reduce mortality associated with a heart disease

10. True or False about the fibric acid derivatives. Gemfibrozil (Lopid) is generally well tolerated

1

TRUE

2

FALSE

3

TRUE

4

TRUE

5

TRUE

6

FALSE

7

FALSE

8

TRUE

9

TRUE

10

TRUE

1. True or False about the bile acid-binding resins. They decrease total cholesterol and LDL

2. True or False about the bile acid-binding resins. They are contraindicated in patients with hypertriglyceridemia

3. True or False about the bile acid-binding resins. When used alone, they do not slow the progression of atherosclerotic lesions

4. True or False about the bile acid-binding resins. They are the drugs of choice for therapy of type II hyperlipidemia when used either alone or in combination with selected agents

5. True or False about nicotinic acid (Niacin). Both triglycerides and LDL cholesterol are reduced by this drug

6. True or False about nicotinic acid (Niacin). The drug acts by directly decreasing the rate of synthesis of apoproteins

7. True or False about nicotinic acid (Niacin). Doses higher than 3 gm/day are no longer used because of possible disturbances of hepatic or pancreatic functions

8. True or False about nicotinic acid (Niacin). Most patients taking this drug experience uncomfortable cutaneous flushing, itching, and/or rashes

9. True or False about the general principles of therapy with lipid-lowering drugs. Therapy with a lipid-lowering drug should be always accompanied by an appropriate diet

10. True or False about the general principles of therapy with lipid-lowering drugs. Lipid-lowering drugs should only be administered after at least 3 months of prior dietary therapy

1	2
TRUE	TRUE
3	4
FALSE	TRUE
5	6
TRUE	FALSE
7	8
TRUE	TRUE
9	10
TRUE	TRUE

1. True or False about the general principles of therapy with lipid-lowering drugs. Some combinations of lipid-lowering drugs are synergistic

2. True or False. The cholesterol synthesis inhibitors increase the rate of clearance of LDL cholesterol from the plasma.

3. True or False. Lovastatin (Mevacor) plus a bile-acid binding resin causes regression of coronary lesions in about one third of treated patients.

4. True or False. The cholesterol synthesis inhibitors are better tolerated than most other lipid-lowering agents.

5. True or False. Selected liver and muscle enzymes should be monitored during the use of any cholesterol synthesis inhibitors because of possible toxic effects.

6. True or False. The bile acid-binding resins act by directly binding cholesterol and facilitating its excretion.

7. True or False. Nicotinic acid (Niacin) acts by increasing the rate of catabolism of VLDL.

8. True or False. Gemfibrozil (Lopid) can cause dizziness and syncope when used with antihypertensives.

9. True or False. Gemfibrozil (Lopid) increases concentrations of HDL cholesterol more than clofibrate (Atromid-S).

10. True or False. The bile acid-binding resins can bind many drugs and vitamins and reduce their absorption.

1 TRUE	2 TRUE
3 TRUE	4 TRUE
5 TRUE	6 FALSE
7 FALSE	8 FALSE
9 TRUE	10 TRUE

1. True or False. When used alone, the bile acid-binding resins are contraindicated in patients with hypertriglyceridemia.

2. True or False. Combinations of lipid-lowering drugs are likely to be synergistic if they work at different steps in the same pathway.

3. True or False. Patients with homozygous familial hypercholesterolemia (type IIa) lack any functional LDL receptors on their hepatocytes.

4. True or False. Effects of drugs in lowering blood cholesterol levels are additive with those of diet.

5. True or False. HMG-CoA reductase inhibiting drugs can cause muscle breakdown, especially when used in combination with a cyclosporine.

6. True or False. Probucol (Lorelco) reduces the risk of atherosclerosis by stimulating the rate of clearance of LDL by receptor-mediated pathways.

7. True or False. Clofibrate (Atromid-S) is generally regarded as superior to gemfibrozil.

8. True or False. Niacin's most common side effects can be reduced by pretreatment with aspirin and/or by taking the drug at the end of meals.

9. True or False. The major side effect of cholestyramine is hepatotoxicity.

10. True or False. The statins are dependent on the presence of LDL receptors on hepatocytes in order to exert their effect.

1	2
TRUE	TRUE
3	4
TRUE	TRUE
5	6
TRUE	FALSE
7	8
FALSE	TRUE
9	10
FALSE	FALSE

1. This drug increases lipoprotein lipase (LPL) activity in adipose tissue

2. This drug both inhibits an enzyme and indirectly enhances clearance of low density lipoproteins (LDL)

3. This drug binds bile acids in the GI tract

4. This drug may block oxidation of low density lipoproteins (LDL)

5. This drug weakly stimulates synthesis of very low density lipoproteins (VLDL)

6. Flushing caused by this drug can be reduced by taking it after meals and/or by pretreatment with aspirin

7. This drug can cause muscle damage, especially when used with any of several drugs including erythromycin

8. This drug decreases blood levels of high density lipoproteins (HDL)

9. This fibric acid derivative increases blood levels of high density lipoproteins (HDL):

10. True or False. Gout is a familial metabolic disease characterized by recurrent episodes of acute arthritis due to deposits of monosodium urate in joints and cartilage.

1 Gemfibrozil (Loprol)	2 Lovastatin (Mevacor)
3 Cholestyramine (Questran)	4 Probucol (Lorelco)
5 Cholestyramine (Questran)	6 Nicotinic acid (niacin)
7 Lovastatin (Mevacor)	8 Probucol (Lorelco)
9 Gemfibrozil (Loprol)	10 TRUE

1. Which drugs is an uricosuric agent

2. Uricosuric drugs are

3. Which drugs used in the treatment of gout acts by preventing the migration of granulocytes

4. Which drugs used in the treatment of gout has as its primary effect the reduction of uric acid synthesis

5. Characteristics of probenecid include

6. True or False. The parathyroid hormone increases serum calcium and decreases serum phosphate.

7. True or False about parathyroid hormone. The parathyroid hormone (PTH) is a single-chain peptide hormone composed of 84 amino acids

8. True or False about parathyroid hormone. The parathyroid hormone increases calcium and phosphate absorption in intestine (by increased 1,25-dihydroxyvitamin D3 production)

9. True or False about parathyroid hormone. The parathyroid hormone increases serum calcium and decreases serum phosphate

10. True or False about parathyroid hormone. The parathyroid hormone increases calcium excretion and decreases phosphate excretion in kidneys

1 Sulfinpyrazone	2 - Probenecid- Sulfinpyrazone- Aspirin (at high dosages)
3 Colchicine	4 Allopurinol
5 - It is useful in the treatment of gout- At appropriate doses, it promotes the excretion of uric acid- The metabolic products of probenecid are uricosuric	6 TRUE
7 TRUE	8 TRUE
9 TRUE	10 FALSE

#		#	
1	True or False about calcitonin. Calcitonin secreted by parafollicular cells of the mammalian thyroid is a single-chain peptide hormone with 32 amino acids	2	True or False about calcitonin. Effects of calcitonin are to lower serum calcium and phosphate by acting on bones and kidneys.
3	True or False about calcitonin. Calcitonin inhibits osteoclastic bone resorption.	4	Mechanism of action of calcitonin is
5	Indications for calcitonin administration are	6	Side effect of calcitonin is
7	Side effect of calcitonin is	8	Glucocorticoid hormones alter bone mineral homeostasis
9	True or False. Estrogens can prevent accelerated bone loss during the immediate postmenopausal period and at least transiently increase bone in the postmenopausal subject.	10	True or False. Vitamin D3 increases serum calcium and phosphate.

1	2
TRUE	TRUE
3	4
TRUE	Raises intracellular cAMP in osteoclasts
5	6
- Hypercalcemia- Paget's disease- Osteoporosis	Tetany
7	8
Hypotension	- By antagonizing vitamin D-stimulated intestinal calcium transport- By stimulating renal calcium excretion- By increasing parathyroid hormone stimulated bone resorption
9	10
TRUE	TRUE

1 Route of administration of vitamin D3 is	2 Side effect of vitamin D3 is
3 Indication of vitamin D3 is	4 Route of administration of 25-hydroxyvitamin D3 (calcifediol) is
5 Indication for 25-hydroxyvitamin D3 (calcifediol) administration is	6 Side effect of 25-hydroxyvitamin D3 (calcifediol) is
7 Indications for 1,25-dihydroxyvitamin D3 (calcitriol) administration are	8 Indication for 1,25-dihydroxyvitamin D3 (calcitriol) administration is
9 True or False about 1,25-dihydroxyvitamin D3 (calcitriol). Calcitriol also raises serum phosphate, though this action is usually not observed early in treatment	10 True or False about 1,25-dihydroxyvitamin D3 (calcitriol). Undergoes enterohepatic circulation

1	2
Oral	Nephrolithiasis

3	4
Hypophosphatemia	Oral

5	6
Failure of vitamin D formation in skin	- Hypercalcemia- Pruritus- GI toxicity

7	8
- Hypocalcemia in chronic renal failure- Vitamin D-dependent rickets- Malabsorption of vitamin D from intestine	Hypophosphatemia

9	10
TRUE	TRUE

1 Route of administration of 1,25-dihydroxyvitamin D3 (calcitriol) is	**2** Commercially available analogs of 1,25-dihydroxyvitamin D3 (calcitriol) are
3 Side effect of dihydrotachysterol is	**4** Route of administration of dihydrotachysterol is
5 Which statements refers to cholecalciferol	**6** Indication for cholecalciferol administration is
7 Route of administration of cholecalciferol is	**8** The unwanted effect of cholecalciferol is
9 The unwanted effect of dihydrotachysterol is	**10** Indication for dihydrotachysterol administration is

1	2
Oral	- Doxercalciferol (Hectoral)- Paricalcitol (Zemplar)

3	4
Hypertension	Oral

5	6
Mechanism of action: 1. Genomic effects 2. Cytoplasmic effects	Malabsorption of vitamin D from intestine

7	8
Oral	CNS toxicity

9	10
CNS toxicity	Hypophosphatemia

1 Conditions associated with hypophosphatemia include	**2** True or False. The long-term effects of hypophosphatemia include proximal muscle weakness and abnormal bone mineralization (osteomalacia).
3 Recommended phosphorus daily allowance is	**4** Interactions with other drugs of phosphorus is
5 Indication for pamidronate administration is	**6** Route of administration of pamidronate is
7 True or False about pamidronate include. Because it causes gastric irritation, pamidronate is not available as an oral preparation	**8** True or False about pamidronate include. Skeletal half-life is 24 h
9 True or False about pamidronate include. Fever and lymphocytopenia are reversible	**10** True or False about pamidronate include. Can be irritable to the esophagus if not washed promptly to the stomach

1 - Primary hyperparathyroidism- Vitamin D deficiency- Idiopathic hypercalciuria	2 TRUE
3 900-1200 mg	4 Calcitonin: increases renal excretion
5 Hypercalcemia	6 Intravenous
7 TRUE	8 FALSE
9 TRUE	10 TRUE

1 Route of administration of alendronate is	2 True or False about alendronate include. Can be irritable to the esophagus if not washed promptly to the stomach
3 True or False about alendronate include. 1st generation biphosphonate	4 True or False about alendronate include. Reduces osteoclast activity without significantly affecting osteoblasts, useful in the treatment of Paget's disease
5 True or False about alendronate include. More potent than EHDP, has a wider therapeutic window	6 Indications of alendronate are
7 Indication for etidronate administration is	8 Indications for etidronate administration are
9 True or False about etidronate. Bioavailability increases with the administered dose	10 True or False about etidronate include. Skeletal half-life is hundreds of days

1	2
Oral	TRUE

3	4
FALSE	TRUE

5	6
TRUE	- Glucocorticoid-induced osteoporosis- Paget's disease- Syndromes of ectopic calcification

7	8
Paget's disease	- Paget's disease- Osteoporosis- Hypercalcemia

9	10
TRUE	TRUE

1. True or False about etidronate include. Bioavailability increases with the administered dose

2. True or False about etidronate include. 2nd generation biphosphonate (amino-biphosphonate)

3. True or False about etidronate include. 1st generation biphosphonate.

4. Unwanted effect of etidronate is:

5. The major causes of hypocalcemia in the adult are

6. The major causes of hypercalcemia in the adult are

7. True or False about calcium. Recommended Ca daily allowance for males: 1. 1-10 years: 800 mg 2. 11-18 years: 1200 mg 3. 19-50 years: 1000 mg 4. > 51 years: 1000 mg

8. True or False about calcium. Ca chloride is very irritating and can cause necrosis if extravasated

9. Indication for calcium administration is

10. Which of the calcium preparations is the most preferable for IV injection

1	2
TRUE	FALSE

3	4
TRUE	Defective bone mineralization

5	6
- Hypoparathyroidism- Vitamin D deficiency- Renal failure and malabsorption	- Hyperparathyroidism- Cancer with or without bone metastases- Hypervitaminosis D

7	8
TRUE	TRUE

9	10
Vitamin D deficiency	Calcium gluconate (0.45 meq calcium/mL)

1 Which of the oral calcium preparations is often the preparation of choice

2 Interactions with other drugs of calcium is

3 True or False about magnesium include. Magnesium is mainly an intracellular cation, and is the fourth most abundant cation in the body

4 True or False about magnesium include. The recommended dietary amounts of magnesium have been set at 6 mg/kg day (350-400 mg)

5 True or False about magnesium include. It is a physiological calcium agonist

6 Recommended magnesium daily allowance is

7 Which of the magnesium preparation is the most preferable for I.V. injection

8 Which of the oral magnesium preparations is often the preparation of choice

9 True or False about fluoride include. Fluoride is effective for the prophylaxis of dental caries

10 True or False about fluoride include. Fluoride is accumulated by bone and teeth, where it may stabilize the hydroxyapatite crystal

1	2
Calcium carbonate (40% calcium)	- Ethanol: decreases absorption- Loop diuretics: increase renal excretion- Glucocorticoids: stimulate renal excretion
3	4
TRUE	TRUE
5	6
FALSE	350-400 mg
7	8
Magnesium chloride	MagneB6 (Mg pidolate / Mg lactate + pyridoxine hydrochloride)
9	10
TRUE	TRUE

1 Recommended fluoride daily allowance is	**2** True or False about gallium nitrate. It is approved by the FDA for the management of hypercalcemia of malignancy
3 True or False about gallium nitrate. This drug acts by inhibiting bone resorption	**4** True or False about gallium nitrate. Because of potential nephrotoxicity, patients should be well-hydrated and have good renal output before starting the infusion
5 True or False about plicamycin (formerly mithramycin). Duration of action is usually several days	**6** True or False about plicamycin (formerly mithramycin). Mechanism of cytotoxic action appears to involve its binding to DNA, possibly through an antibiotic-Mg^{2+} complex.
7 Unwanted effects of plicamycin (formerly mithramycin) are	**8** Unwanted effect of plicamycin (formerly mithramycin) is
9 Indication for plicamycin (formerly mithramycin) administration is	**10** Route of administration of plicamycin is

1	2
1.5-4 mg	TRUE

3	4
TRUE	TRUE

5	6
TRUE	TRUE

7	8
Fractures	Myelosuppression

9	10
- Testicular cancers refractory to standard treatment- Paget's disease- Hypercalcemia of malignancy	Intravenous

1. Mineralocorticoid effects cause

2. Which synthetic steroids shows predominantly mineralocorticoid action?

3. The major mineralocorticoids are

4. True or False about spironolactone. Spironolactone reverses many of the manifestations of aldosteronism

5. True or False about spironolactone. Spironilactone is also an androgen antagonist and as such is used in the treatment of hirsutism in wormen

6. True or False about spironolactone. Spironolactone is useful as a diuretic

7. True or False about diuretics. Carbonic anhydrase inhibition leads to increased reabsorption of NaHCO3

8. True or False about diuretics. Loop diuretics decrease Na+ reabsorption at the loop of Henle by competing for the Cl- site on the Na+/K+/2Cl cotransporter

9. True or False about diuretics. In general, the potency of a diuretic is determined by where it acts in the renal tubule

10. True or False about diuretics. Hydrochlorothiazide decreases urinary calcium excretion

1	2
Increased Na retension and K excretion	Fludrocortisone
3	4
Hydrocortisone	TRUE
5	6
TRUE	TRUE
7	8
FALSE	TRUE
9	10
TRUE	TRUE

1 The drug inhibits the ubiquitous enzyme carbonic anhydrase	**2** The drug acts by competitively blocking NaCl cotransporters in the distal tubule
3 The drug acts at the proximal tubule	**4** The drug acts by competing with aldosterone for its cytosolic receptors
5 The drug is a potassium-sparing diuretic that blocks Na+ channels in the collecting tubules	**6** Chronic use of this drug can lead to distal tubular hypertrophy, which may reduce its diuretic effect
7 The drug has a steroid-like structure which is responsible for its anti-androgenic effect	**8** Sustained use of this drug results in increased plasma urate concentrations
9 The drug can be used to treat glaucoma	**10** The drug can cause ototoxicity

1 Acetazolamide (Diamox)	2 Hydrochlorothiazide (HydroDiuril)
3 Acetazolamide (Diamox)	4 Spironolactone (Aldactone)
5 Amiloride (Midamor)	6 Furosemide (Lasix)
7 Spironolactone (Aldactone)	8 Furosemide (Lasix)
9 Acetazolamide (Diamox)	10 Furosemide (Lasix)

1	2
The drug acts only on the lumenal side of renal tubules	The drug can promote sodium loss in patients with low (e.g., 40 ml/min) glomerular filtration rates
3	4
The drug can be used to treat nephrogenic diabetes insipidus	The drug is sometimes part of fixed-dose combinations used to treat essential hypertension
5	6
The drug should never be administered to patients taking potassium supplements	The drug decreases calcium excretion in urine
7	8
The drug acts by competitively blocking the Na+/K+/2Cl- cotransporter	The drug acts at the proximal tubule
9	10
The drug acts in the distal convoluted tubule	The drug acts in the collecting tubules

1	2
Furosemide (Lasix)	Furosemide (Lasix)

3	4
Hydrochlorothiazide (HydroDiuril)	Hydrochlorothiazide (HydroDiuril)-Amiloride (Midamor)

5	6
Amiloride (Midamor)	Hydrochlorothiazide (HydroDiuril)

7	8
Loop diuretics	Carbonic anhydrase inhibitors

9	10
Thiazide diuretics	Potassium-sparing diuretics

1 The drug is the most potent diuretic	**2** The drug acts by competitively blocking the NaCl cotransporter
3 The drug inhibits sodium and chloride transport in the cortical thick ascending limb and the early distal tubule	**4** The drug can cause ototoxicity
5 The drug blocks the sodium/potassium/chloride cotransporter in the thick ascending loop of Henle	**6** The drug is one of the most potent diuretics
7 The drug is usually given in combination with a thiazide diuretic	**8** True or False about diuretics. Furosemide (Lasix) can increase the likelihood of digitalis toxicity
9 True or False about diuretics. Chlorthalidone (Hygroton) can decrease the excretion of lithium	**10** True or False about diuretics. Ibuprofen can increase the antihypertensive effect of chlorthalidone

1	2
Loop diuretics	Thiazide diuretics

3	4
Hydrochlorothiazide (Hydrodiuril)	Furosemide (Lasix)

5	6
Furosemide (Lasix)	Furosemide (Lasix)

7	8
Amiloride (Midamor)	TRUE

9	10
TRUE	FALSE

1
True or False about diuretics. Chlorthalidone has a longer duration of action than furosemide

2
The drug is the least potent diuretic

3
These agents must be given parenterally because they are not absorbed when given orally

4
These drugs may be used in the treatment of recurrent calcium nephrolithiasis

5
Furosemide (Lasix) acts at this nephron site

6
Metolazone (Mykrox) acts at this nephron site

7
Acetazolamide (Diamox) acts at this nephron site

8
Spironolactone (Aldactone) acts at this nephron site

9
Amiloride (Midamone) acts at this nephron site

10
The drug competitively blocks chloride channels and prevents movement of sodium, potassium, and chloride into the renal tubular cells

1	2
TRUE	Potassium-sparing diuretics
3	4
Osmotic diuretics	Loop diuretics
5	6
Ascending thick limb of the loop of Henle	Distal convoluted tubule
7	8
Proximal convoluted tubule	Collecting duct
9	10
Collecting duct	Furosemide (Lasix)

1. The drug acts by affecting the tubular fluid composition in a non-receptor mediated fashion

2. The drug is a blood substitute having haemodynamical activity

3. This drug is a desintoxicative plasma substitute

4. This drug is a controller of water-salt and acid-basic state

5. What does the term "antibiotics" mean

6. Minimal duration of antibacterial treatment usually is

7. Rational anti-microbial combination is used to

8. Mechanisms of bacterial resistance to anti-microbial agents are

9. True or False. The statement, that some microorganisms can develop alternative metabolic pathways for rendering reactions inhibited by the drug

10. Bactericidal effect is

1 Mannitol (Osmitrol)	2 Polyglucinum
3 Haemodesum	4 "Disolum", "Trisolum"
5 Substances produced by some microorganisms and their synthetic analogues that selectively kill or inhibit the growth of another microorganisms	6 Not less than 5 days
7 - Provide synergism when microorganisms are not effectively eradicated with a single agent alone- Provide broad coverage- Prevent the emergence of resistance	8 - Active transport out of a microorganism or/and hydrolysis of an agent via enzymes produced by a microorganism- Modification of a drug's target- Reduced uptake by a microorganism
9 TRUE	10 Destroying of bacterial cells

1 Which roups of antibiotics demonstrates a bactericidal effect?	2 Bacteristatic effect is
3 Which groups of antibiotics demonstrates a bacteristatic effect	4 Which antibiotics contains a beta-lactam ring in their chemical structure
5 Drug belonging to antibiotics-macrolides	6 Drug belonging to antibiotics-carbapenems
7 Drug belonging to antibiotics-monobactams	8 Drug belongs to antibiotics-cephalosporins
9 Drug belonging to lincozamides	10 Drug belonging to antibiotics-tetracyclines

1	2
Penicillins	Inhibition of bacterial cell division
3	4
Macrolides	- Penicillins- Cephalosporins- Carbapenems and monobactams
5	6
Erythromycin	Imipinem
7	8
Aztreonam	Cefaclor
9	10
Lincomycin	Doxycycline

1 Exemples of aminoglycosides	2 Drug belonging to nitrobenzene derivative
3 Drug belonging to glycopeptides	4 Antibiotics inhibiting the bacterial cell wall synthesis are
5 Antibiotic inhibiting bacterial RNA synthesis is	6 Antibiotics altering permeability of cell membranes are
7 All of the following antibiotics inhibit the protein synthesis in bacterial cells	8 Biosynthetic penicillins are effective against
9 Which drugs is a gastric acid resistant	10 Which drugs is penicillinase resistant

1	2
- Gentamycin- Streptomycin- Neomycin	Chloramphenicol

3	4
Vancomycin	Beta-lactam antibiotics

5	6
Rifampin	Polymyxins

7	8
- Macrolides- Aminoglycosides- Tetracyclines	Gram-positive and gram-negative cocci, Corynebacterium diphtheria, spirochetes, Clostridium gangrene

9	10
Penicillin V	Oxacillin

1 All of the following drugs demonstrate a prolonged effect	**2** Mechanism of penicillins' antibacterial effect is
3 Beta-lactamase inhibitor for co-administration with penicillins	**4** Cephalosporines are drugs of choice for treatment of
5 Carbapenems are effective against	**6** All of the following antibiotics are macrolides
7 Tetracyclins have following unwanted effects	**8** Drug belonging to antibiotics-aminoglycosides
9 Aminoglycosides are effective against	**10** Aminoglycosides have the following unwanted effects

1 - Procain penicillin- Bicillin-1- Bicillin-5	**2** Inhibition of transpeptidation in the bacterial cell wall
3 - Clavulanic acid- Sulbactam- Tazobactam	**4** Gram-negative and gram-positive microorganism infections, if penicillins have no effect
5 Broad-spectum	**6** - Erythromycin- Clarithromycin- Roxythromycin
7 - Irritation of gastrointestinal mucosa, phototoxicity- Hepatotoxicity, anti-anabolic effect- Dental hypoplasia, bone deformities	**8** Gentamycin
9 Broad-spectrum, except anaerobic microorganisms and viruses	**10** Ototoxicity, nephrotoxicity

1. Characteristics of chloramphenicol

2. Chloramphenicol has the following unwanted effects

3. Characteristics of lincozamides

4. Lincozamides have the following unwanted effect

5. Characteristics of vancomicin

6. Vancomicin has the following unwanted effects

7. Which drugs is used for systemic and deep mycotic infections treatment:

8. Which drugs is used for dermatomycosis treatment

9. Which drugs is used for candidiasis treatment

10. The following antifungal drugs are antibiotics

1	2
Broad-spectum. Demonstrates a bactericidal effect.	Pancytopenia

3	4
Influence mainly the anaerobic organisms, Gram positive cocci.	Pseudomembranous colitis

5	6
It is a glycopeptide, inhibits cell wall synthesis and is active only against Gram-positive bacteria.	"Red neck" syndrome, phlebitis

7	8
Amphotericin B	Griseofulvin

9	10
Myconazol	Myconazol

1

Mechanism of Amphotericin B action is

2

Azoles have an antifungal effect because of

3

Which drugs alters permeability of Candida cell membranes

4

Amfotericin B has the following unwanted effects

5

Drug belonging to antibiotics having a polyene structure

6

The following drugs demonstrate a fungicidal effect

7

The following drug do not demonstrate a fungicidal effect

8

Characteristics of polyenes are

9

Characteristics of polyenes are not

10

Characteristics of Amfotericin B are

1	2
Alteration of cell membrane permeability	Reduction of ergosterol synthesis
3	4
Nystatin	Renal impairment, anemia
5	6
Nystatin	- Terbinafin- Ketoconazole- Myconazol
7	8
Amfotericin B	- Alter the structure and functions of cell membranes- Broad-spectrum- Nephrotoxicity, hepatotoxicity
9	10
Fungicidal effect	- Used for systemic mycosis treatment- Poor absorption from the gastro-intestinal tract- Influences the permeability of fungus cell membrane

1
Characteristics of Amfotericin B are not

2
Sulfonamides are effective against

3
Mechanism of sulfonamides' antibacterial effect is

4
Combination of sulfonamides with trimethoprim

5
Sulfonamide potency is decreased in case of co-administration with

6
The following measures are necessary for prevention of sulfonamide precipitation and crystalluria

7
Resorptive sulfonamides have the following unwanted effects on blood system

8
Mechanism of Trimethoprim' action is

9
Sulfonamides have the following unwanted effects

10
The drug, which is effective against mycobacteria only

1 Does not demonstrate nephrotoxicity	2 - Bacteria and Chlamidia- Actinomyces- Protozoa
3 Inhibition of dihydropteroate synthase	4 Increases the antimicrobial activity
5 Local anesthetics – derivatives of paraaminobenzoic acid	6 Taking of drinks with alkaline pH
7 - Hemolytic anemia- Thrombocytopenia- Granulocytopenia	8 Inhibition of dihydropteroate reductase
9 - Hematopoietic disturbances- Crystalluria- Nausea, vomiting and diarrhea	10 Isoniazid

1	2
The antimycobacterial drug belonging to first-line agents	The antimycobacterial drug, belonging to second-line agents
3	4
The antimycobacterial drug, belonging to antibiotics	Mechanism of Izoniazid action is
5	6
Mechanism of Rifampin action is	Mechanism of Cycloserine action is
7	8
Mechanism of Streptomycin action is	Rifampin has the following unwanted effect
9	10
Isoniazid has following unwanted effect	Ethambutol has the following unwanted effect

1 Isoniazid	2 PAS
3 Rifampin	4 Inhibition of mycolic acids synthesis
5 Inhibition of DNA dependent RNA polymerase	6 Inhibition of cell wall synthesis
7 Inhibition of protein synthesis	8 Flu-like syndrome, tubular necrosis
9 Hepatotoxicity, peripheral neuropathy	10 Retrobulbar neuritis with red-green color blindness

1. Streptomycin has the following unwanted effect

2. Mechanism of aminosalicylic acid action is

3. The following agents are the first-line antimycobacterial drugs

4. The following antimycobacterial drugs have a bactericidal effect

5. Combined chemotherapy of tuberculosis is used to

6. Antibacterial drug – a nitrofurane derivative

7. Antibacterial drug – a nitroimidazole derivative

8. Antibacterial drug – a quinolone derivative

9. Antibacterial drug – a fluoroquinolone derivative

10. The indications for nitrofuranes

1	2
Ototoxicity, nephrotoxicity	Inhibition of folate synthesis

3	4
- Rifampin- Isoniazid- Streptomycin	- Streptomycin- Rifampin- Isoniazid

5	6
Decrease mycobacterium drug-resistance	Nitrofurantoin

7	8
Metronidazole	Nalidixic acid

9	10
Ciprofloxacin	Infections of urinary and gastro-intestinal tracts

1	2
The unwanted effects of nitrofuranes	The indications for Metronidazole

3	4
The unwanted effects of Metronidazole	The mechanism of fluoroquinolones' action is

5	6
Fluoroquinolones are active against	The unwanted effects of fluoroquinolones

7	8
The indications for fluoroquinolones	The drug of choice for syphilis treatment is

9	10
The drug used for malaria chemoprophylaxis and treatment	The drug used for amoebiasis treatment

1 - Nausea, vomiting- Allergic reactions- Hemolytic anemia	2 Intra-abdominal infections, vaginitis enterocolitis
3 Nausea, vomiting, diarrhea, stomatitis	4 Inhibition of DNA gyrase
5 Variety of Gram-negative and positive microorganisms, including Mycoplasmas and Chlamidiae	6 Headache, dizziness, insomnia
7 Infections of the urinary and respiratory tract, bacterial diarrhea	8 Penicillin
9 Chloroquine	10 Iodoquinol

1. The drug used for trichomoniasis treatment	2. The drug used for toxoplasmosis treatment
3. The drug used for balantidiasis treatment	4. The drug used for leishmaniasis treatment
5. The antimalarial drug belonging to 8-aminoquinoline derivatives	6. The following antimalarial drugs are 4-quinoline derivatives
7. The following antimalarial drugs are not 4-quinoline derivatives	8. The antimalarial drug belonging to pyrimidine derivat
9. The drug used for trypanosomosis treatment	10. The antimalarial drug having a gametocidal effect

1	2
Metronidazole	Pyrimethamine
3	4
Tetracycline	Sodium stibogluconate
5	6
Primaquine	- Chloroquine- Mefloquine- Amodiaquine
7	8
Primaquine	Pyrimethamine
9	10
Melarsoprol	Primaquine

1 The following antimalarial drugs influence blood schizonts	2 The following antimalarial drugs do not influence blood schizonts
3 The antimalarial drug influencing tissue schisonts	4 The group of antibiotics having an antimalarial effect
5 The amebecide drug for the treatment of an asymptomatic intestinal form of amebiasis	6 The drugs for the treatment of an intestinal form of amebiasis
7 The drug for the treatment of a hepatic form of amebiasis	8 The luminal amebecide drug
9 The drug of choice for the treatment of extraluminal amebiasis	10 The drug, blocking acetylcholine transmission at the myoneural junction of helminthes

1	2
- Mefloquine- Chloroquine- Quinidine	Primaquine

3	4
Primaquine	Tetracyclins

5	6
Diloxanide	Metronidazole and diloxanide

7	8
Metronidazole or emetine	Diloxanide

9	10
Metronidazole	Piperazine

1 Niclosamide mechanism of action	2 Praziquantel mechanism of action
3 Piperazine mechanism of action	4 The drug, a salicylamide derivative
5 Mebendazole mechanism of action	6 The drug, inhibiting oxidative phosphorylation in some species of helminthes
7 The drug for neurocysticercosis treatment	8 The drug for nematodosis (roundworm invasion) treatment
9 The drug for cestodosis (tapeworm invasion) treatment	10 The drug for trematodosis (fluke invasion) treatment

1 Inhibiting oxidative phosphorylation in some species of helminthes	2 Increasing cell membrane permeability for calcium, resulting in paralysis, dislodgement and death of helminthes
3 Blocking acetylcholine transmission at the myoneural junction and paralysis of helminthes	4 Niclosamide
5 Inhibiting microtubule synthesis in helminthes and irreversible impairment of glucose uptake	6 Niclosamide
7 Praziquante	8 Pyrantel
9 Praziquantel	10 Bithionol

1	2
The drug, a benzimidazole derivative	The broad spectrum drug for cestodosis, trematodosis and cycticercosis treatment
3	**4**
The drug for ascaridosis and enterobiosis treatment	The drug for strongiloidosis treatment
5	**6**
The drug for echinococcosis treatment	The following antiviral drugs are the analogs of nucleosides
7	**8**
The drug, a derivative of adamantane	The drug, a derivative of pyrophosphate
9	**10**
The drug, inhibiting viral DNA synthesis	The drug, inhibiting uncoating of the viral RNA

1	2
Mebendazole	Praziquantel
3	4
Pyrantel	Ivermectin
5	6
Mebendazole or Albendazole	Saquinavir
7	8
Rimantadine	Foscarnet
9	10
Acyclovir	Rimantadine

1. The drug, inhibiting viral reverse transcriptase	2. The drug, inhibiting viral proteases
3. The drug of choice for herpes and cytomegalovirus infection treatment	4. The drug which belongs to nonnucleoside reverse transcriptase inhibitors
5. The following antiviral drugs are antiretroviral agents	6. The drug used for influenza A prevention
7. The drug used for HIV infection treatment, a derivative of nucleosides	8. The antiviral drug which belongs to endogenous proteins
9. The drug which belongs to nucleoside reverse transcriptase inhibitors	10. The following antiviral drugs are anti-influenza agents

1	2
Zidovudine	Saquinavir

3	4
Acyclovir	Nevirapine

5	6
- Zidovudine- Zalcitabine- Didanozine	Rimantadine

7	8
Zidovudine	Interferon alfa

9	10
Didanosine	- Amantadine- Interferons- Rimantadine

1	2
The unwanted effects of zidovudine	The unwanted effects of intravenous acyclovir infusion

3	4
The drug that can induce peripheral neuropathy and oral ulceration	The unwanted effects of didanozine

5	6
The unwanted effects of indinavir	The drug that can induce nausea, diarrhea, abdominal pain and rhinitis

7	8
The following effects are disadvantages of anticancer drugs	Rational combination of anticancer drugs is used to

9	10
The anticancer alkylating drug, a derivative of chloroethylamine	The anticancer alkylating drug, a derivative of ethylenimine

1	2
Anemia, neutropenia, nausea, insomnia	Renal insufficiency, tremors, delerium

3	4
Zalcitabine	Peripheral neuropathy, pancreatitis, diarrhea, hyperuricemia

5	6
Nephrolithiasis, nausea, hepatotoxicity	Saquinavir

7	8
- Low selectivity to cancer cells- Depression of bone marrow- Depression of immune system	Provide synergism resulting from the use of anticancer drugs with different mechanisms combination

9	10
Cyclophosphamide	Thiotepa

1. The group of hormonal drugs used for cancer treatment	2. The anticancer alkylating drug, a derivative of alkylsulfonate
3. The anticancer drug of plant origin	4. Action mechanism of alkylating agents is
5. The anticancer drug, a pyrimidine antagonist	6. Methotrexate is
7. The antibiotic for cancer chemotherapy	8. Fluorouracil belongs to
9. The action mechanism of anticancer drugs belonging to plant alkaloids	10. General contraindications for anticancer drugs are

1	2
Glucocorticoids and gonadal hormones	Busulfan
3	4
Vincristine	Producing carbonium ions altering DNA structure
5	6
Fluorouracil	A folic acid antagonist
7	8
Doxorubicin	Antimetabolites
9	10
Mitotic arrest at a metaphase	- Depression of bone marrow- Acute infections- Severe hepatic and/or renal insufficiency

1 Action mechanism of methotrexate is	2 The anticancer drug belonging to inorganic metal complexes
3 The indication for estrogens in oncological practice	4 Enzyme drug used for acute leukemia treatment
5 The following drugs are derivatives of nitrosoureas	6 The group of drugs used as subsidiary medicines in cancer treatment
7 Estrogen inhibitor	8 Antiandrogen drug
9 The drug belonging to aromatase inhibitors	10 The drug belonging to gonadotropin-releasing hormone agonists

1	2
Inhibition of dihydrofolate reductase	Cisplatin

3	4
Cancer of prostate	Dihydrofolate reductase

5	6
- Carmustine- Lomustine- Semustine	- Cytoprotectors- Bone marrow growth factors- Antimetastatic agents

7	8
Tamoxifen	Flutamide

9	10
Anastrozole	Leuprolide

www.ingramcontent.com/pod-product-compliance
Lightning Source LLC
Chambersburg PA
CBHW080954170526
45158CB00010B/2797